100 BEST

WEIGHT-LOSS
TIPS

OTHER BOOKS BY THE AUTHOR:

WALK, DON'T RUN. Philadelphia: Medical Manor Press, 1979.

THE DOCTOR'S WALKING BOOK. New York: Ballantine Books, a Division of Random House Books, 1980.

DIETWALK®: THE DOCTOR'S FAST 3-DAY SUPERDIET. Philadelphia: Medical Manor Books®, 1983.
Pocket Books® Edition, Simon & Schuster, New York, 1987.

WALK, DON'T DIE. Philadelphia: Medical Manor Books®, 1986.
Bart Books Edition: New York, 1988.

WALK TO WIN: THE EASY 4-DAY DIET & FITNESS PLAN. Philadelphia: Medical Manor Books®, 1990.

DIET-STEP: 20 GRAMS/20 MINUTES-FOR WOMEN ONLY! Philadelphia: Medical Manor Books®, 2002.

POWER DIET-STEP: DR. STUTMAN'S 21-DAY POWER WEIGHT-LOSS & FITNESS PLAN. Philadelphia: Medical Manor Books®, 2005.

DIET-STEP: 30/30-FOR SENIORS ONLY. Philadelphia: Medical Manor Books®, 2005.

100 BEST FITNESS TIPS. Philadelphia: Medical Manor Books®, 2005.

Medical Manor Books® are available at special quantity discounts for sales promotions, premiums, fund raising or educational use.
Book excerpts can also be created to fit special needs. For details write to: Special Markets Dept. Medical Manor Books®
3501 Newberry Rd. Philadelphia, PA 19154.
Phone: 1-800-DIETING (343-8464)
E-mail: info@medicalmanorbooks.com
Web: www.medicalmanorbooks.com

100 BEST

WEIGHT-LOSS
TIPS

By
Fred A. Stutman, M.D.

Medical Manor Books®
Philadelphia, Pa

100 BEST WEIGHT-LOSS TIPS

Copyright© 2005 by Fred A. Stutman, M.D.

MEDICAL MANOR BOOKS® is the registered trademark of Manor House Publications, Inc. REG. U.S. PAT. OFF.

DR. WALK® is the registered trademark of Dr. Stutman's Diet & Fitness Newsletter. REG. U.S. PAT. OFF.

DIET-STEP® is the registered trademark of Dr. Stutman's Weight-Loss and Fitness program. REG. U.S. PAT. OFF.

FIT-STEP® is the registered trademark of Dr. Stutman's Fitness Walking Program. REG. U.S. PAT. OFF.

TRIM-STEP® is the registered trademark of Dr. Stutman's Strength Training and Stretching Program. REG. U.S. PAT. OFF.

POWER DIET-STEP® is the registered trademark of Dr. Stutman's 21-Day Power Weight Loss & Fitness Plan.

Library of Congress Cataloging-in-Publication Data

Stutman, Fred A.
100 best weight-loss tips / by Fred A. Stutman.— 1st ed.
p. cm.
ISBN 0-934232-20-2 — ISBN 0-934232-19-9
1. Weight loss. I. Title: One hundred best weight-loss tips. II. Title.
RM222.2.S877 2005
613.2'5—dc22   2004050481

First Edition 2005
Manufactured in the United States of America

To

Suzanne

Geoffrey, Samantha, Alana, Rain

&

Sparkey

AUTHOR'S CAUTION

IT IS ESSENTIAL THAT YOU CONSULT YOUR OWN PHYSICIAN BEFORE FOLLOWING ANY OF THE 100 BEST WEIGHT-LOSS TIPS.

Fred A. Stutman, M.D.

ACKNOWLEDGEMENTS

EDITOR: Suzanne Stutman, Ph.D.

EDITORIAL STAFF: Patricia McGarvey, Eileen Bedara, Mary Ann Johnston, Linda Quinn, Sheryl Bartkus, Pattie Hartigan, Kathy Bradley

PERMISSIONS: Physicians' Health Bulletin; Sorosh Roshan, M.D., President, International Health Awareness Network; J & J Snack Foods, Inc.; Carol Verdi, M.D., Temple University Family Practice Physician; Vera Tweed, Let's Live Magazine; Alan Caruba, Editor, www.bookviews.com; Kirkus Reports; James A. Cox, Editor-in-Chief, The Midwest Book Review

MEDICAL DICTATION: Accu-Med Transcription Service

TYPOGRAPHY & GRAPHIC DESIGN: Alexander E. Shin, Sir Speedy Graphic Design

BOOK MANUFACTURING: Thomson-Shore, Inc.

COVER DESIGN: Geralynne Slowe

PUBLISHER: Medical Manor Books®

TABLE OF CONTENTS

IV. PROTEIN TIPS

V. FAT TIPS

VI. GREAT WEIGHT-LOSS TIPS

VII. SECRET GET-SLIM TIPS

VIII. CALORIE - BLASTING TIPS

IX. DIET-STEP® TIPS

X. POWER FAT-BURNING TIPS

INTRODUCTION

Save your money. Throw away your diet books. Quit your weekly weigh-ins at the neighborhood diet center. Stop trying unhealthy, low-carbohydrate and other fad diets that invariably result in rebound weight gain. *100 Best Weight-Loss Tips* are all you ever need to lose weight easily and maintain your ideal weight safely. There are no formal diet plans to follow, no complicated recipes to prepare and no nasty-tasting diet shakes to gulp down. And there are no strenuous exercises to engage in and no expensive fitness clubs to join. *100 Best Weight-Loss Tips* provides a dynamic course of action for those interested in losing weight quickly and safely. This new book translates for the reader the science behind diet and nutrition and presents suggestions for healthy food choices in language which is concise and easy to understand.

100 Best Weight Loss Tips give you all of the necessary building blocks to follow for a lifetime, promoting healthy eating habits and a safe and easy permanent weight-loss system. There is no need to follow unsafe low-carbohydrate diets that deprive you of healthy, good tasting nutritious foods. These unhealthy diets not only fill up your body's fat cells with extra pounds of fat, but they also can clog your arteries with cholesterol, which increases your risk of heart attacks and strokes. Kidney and liver damage have also been reported to occur in some people who have been on extended low carbohydrate diets. Low carbohydrate diets are not only extremely dangerous to your health, but invariably lead to rebound weight gain once they are stopped.
.

The diet business, ranging from diet centers, spas, health clubs and diet foods, generated more than 38 billion dollars in revenues in 2004. This figure is comparable to the revenues of the casino industry, which is just a different form of gambling. Consumer reports polled 95,000 subscribers who tried to lose weight over the last three to five years. Over 19,000 subscribers used commercially supervised programs, and the rest tried to lose weight on their own. The results of both groups were similar in that dieters lost an average of 10 to 12 pounds while on their respective diets. The discouraging news, however, is that most of the respondents to this survey regained almost one-half of their weight loss in the first three to six months after ending the diet program. After a period of two years, these same dieters regained 2/3 of the weight that they had originally lost. Many of these commercial diet programs cost an average of $75.00 per week—a pretty hefty price to pay for temporary weight loss.

This series of weight-loss tips has been thoroughly researched for medical authenticity and is safe and effective and provides you with a unique, easy-to-follow weight-loss system. All you need to do is follow the *100 Best Weight-Loss Tips* every day and you will lose weight easily, safely, and permanently without the health dangers posed by unsafe low-carbohydrate and other fad diets. You won't experience any rebound weight gain and most importantly you'll improve your health and add years to your life. These tips were designed with you in mind. Boost your energy level, lose weight, and get firm and fit with actually very little effort on your part. You will feel better, look younger, be thinner, get firmer, and lose weight with each and every weight-loss tip that you follow. The weight you lose will stay lost forever.

I.
CARB TIPS

TIP # 1
LOW CARB DIETS ARE DANGEROUS!

The low carbohydrate diet craze, which is essentially a high-fat, high-protein, low-carbohydrate diet, is a component of practically every diet book that has been on the market for the past ten years. The first question that comes to mind is, "Then, how do people lose weight on these low-carbohydrate, high-fat diets?" For example, most of the diets say that you can have bacon and eggs for breakfast, hot dogs for lunch, and a juicy steak for dinner. Sounds tempting, doesn't it? They also tell you that you can't have any, or, at the very least, minimal amounts of carbohydrates with each meal; for instance, no vegetables, fruits, cereals, breads, potatoes, pasta, etc. Sounds unappetizing and unhealthy, doesn't it? It certainly is.

The simple fact is that you do lose weight initially on these very low-carbohydrate, high-fat, high-protein diets; however, most of the initial weight-loss is *water weight-loss,* due to a metabolic process called *ketosis,* which, in fact, is a condition found in unhealthy people (for example, those with diabetes and kidney disease), and not in healthy people. Once the body gets rid of this water, it starts burning fat, which is left over – which, in itself, is a good thing; however, the downside is that this abnormal process of ketosis also begins to burn the body's protein (muscle tissue). This actually is a very bad thing. By attempting to burn protein as a source of fuel for energy, the body is actually breaking down one of the most important elements in the body that is used to sustain life (building and repairing the body's tissues, cells, and organs).

The fact that a substance called ketones appears in your urine (a by-product of this abnormal process called ketosis) shows you clear evidence that your body is breaking down its muscle tissue. This is one of the reasons that fatigue and general weakness have been reported as early side effects of this completely unhealthy diet.

Also, kidney and liver damage may result if too much of the body's protein is broken down in these unhealthy, low-carbohydrate diets.

In ketosis, fatty acids are broken down to form ketones and acetones, which the body can then use as fuel. Unfortunately, this results in the loss of sodium and potassium from the body, which are vital minerals essential for health. Even levels of thyroid hormone decrease and your metabolism slows down to conserve energy, which, in turn, slows the process of weight-loss. During this process of ketosis, the blood cholesterol goes up, which, in itself, is a dangerous condition.

While the body is breaking down fat to form ketones for energy, it must consume some of its muscle tissue (protein) to meet the energy needs of the brain and nervous system. Since the brain and nervous system use approximately two-thirds of the glucose present in the body, ketones cannot replace glucose for many of the brain's functions. This, in turn, can affect the brain adversely, since protein must be broken down to form amino acids, which can then be converted to glucose. If this is not done in a timely fashion, then the brain's blood supply of glucose is limited, resulting in temporary and/or permanent neurological damage.

As you can see, this is a dangerous way to diet and is not a healthy type of diet to remain on for any period of time. In addition, once this diet is stopped, rapid weight gain resumes, since the body has been depleted of carbohydrates, water and nutrients. The hunger center (appestat) in the brain increases your appetite, and you usually begin to consume massive quantities of carbohydrates to alleviate the adverse effects of this diet.

TIP # 2
LOW CARB DIETS ARE INSANE!

An article reported at the American College of Preventive Medicine's annual meeting (ACPM 2004: Session 33; February 21, 2004), stated that "Low carbohydrate diets, such as the Atkins and the South Beach Diet, are based on a premise that is so utterly wrong as to be insane," according to David L. Katz, M.D., MPH, from the Yale Preventive Medicine Research Center in New Haven, Connecticut. This article was reported in the Medscape Medical News Report 2004.

This article went on to say that any diet that doesn't correct energy imbalance, for example more calories ingested than calories burned, would not stand the test of time. This article further cautioned that the food industry is responding to the low-carb frenzy with many new low-carb products, including low-carb beers, breads, cereals, and even marshmallows. They also claimed that many low-fat products are just as bad, since, like the low-carb products, they contain far too many calories. The article warned that using the glycemic index to select foods, as recommended in many low-carb diet books, often leads to ridiculous choices. For example, ice cream has a lower glycemic index than carrots. Hello!

These low-carbohydrate, high-fat, high-protein diets promise weight-loss by utilizing a diet that has more than 60% of its calories coming from fat. In addition, these diets put no restriction on the type of fat, whether it's saturated, unsaturated, or fat that's high in cholesterol. These foods consist of high saturated fat meat sources, such as hamburger, steak, bacon, sausage, and ham, including turkey and chicken with the skin left intact, and high-fat milk products, such as whole milk, cheeses, heavy cream, hard cheeses, and eggs. They also encourage consumption of high-fat salad dressings with saturated oils. They unfortunately restrict nutritious fruits, vegetables, cereals, beans, and breads, whether refined or whole-wheat, and desserts and sweets.

These diets have been popularized for the past 10-15 years and have shown little scientific evidence of their effectiveness or their safety. The most recent data on these diets has shown that any weight- loss that occurs is primarily due to the consumption of fewer calories, not fewer carbs. However, in most cases, weight gain invariably occurs since these diets are basically high in calories, as well as high in fat and protein. So you're actually getting a double whammy here: fat build-up in your arteries and fat build-up in your face, abdomen, buttocks, and thighs. And if this wasn't bad enough, then think of the potential damage that these diets can do to your kidneys from the abnormal state of ketosis that results from these low-carb diets.

These rapid-weight-loss, low-carbohydrate, high-fat, high-protein diets have what is called "rebound weight gain." This occurs after the initial weight-loss, which results from fat and protein breakdown, which was used for energy production (fuel). The body's carbohydrate stores then become depleted because of the very low intake of carbohydrates in these diets, and thus there is limited availability of carbohydrates to be burned as a fuel. Unfortunately, these low stores of carbohydrates are designated to be the very first type of calories to be burned as fuel in our normal metabolism.

Once your body becomes aware that it is carbohydrate-depleted, by exhibiting the symptoms of fatigue, malaise, muscle cramps, and decreased urine output, which occurs after the initial weight-loss, then your brain's control center receives stress signals from all of your body's cells suffering from carbohydrate depletion. Your brain's hunger center then has no other option but to set you off on a carbohydrate binge to replace the carbohydrate depletion felt by all of the body's cells.

What follows is rebound weight gain until your sweet tooth gets satisfied and you begin to resume your former unhealthy diet of excess fat and low carbohydrates. Not a pretty picture, is it? And yet, over 75% of the commercially available diet books work on this abnormal metabolic process principle.

Since this diet is primarily animal protein, you are shorting yourself on vitamins, minerals, antioxidants, phytochemicals, essential fatty acids, and fiber. These important nutrients, which are primarily found in plant foods (vegetables, grains, and fruits), have been proven to protect against and prevent heart disease, cancer, strokes, and a variety of other degenerative diseases. The more animal fat that you consume with this diet, the more you increase your risk of cardiovascular and cerebrovascular disease, in other words, strokes or heart attacks. This is caused by the elevation of blood fats caused by this diet, particularly cholesterol and a protein/fat combination called lipoproteins.

TIP # 3
BAD CARBS

There is no clear evidence that low carbohydrate diets are better than low-fat diets in helping people to lose weight. These low- carbohydrate diets can promote short-term weight-loss; however, weight gain rebound occurs in over 90% of the people who go off of these boring, high-fat, high-protein, dangerous diets. In most cases, these individuals gain back almost all of their original weight, with an added 20% bonus of additional pounds.

Your body converts all of the carbohydrates that you eat into sugar (glucose), which our body's cells use as fuel. When these glucose molecules pass from the intestines into the bloodstream, the organ known as the pancreas produces insulin, which tells the body's cells to absorb the glucose. Once the cells (skin, internal organs, tissues, muscles, fat, and others) absorb the glucose, then the insulin levels return to normal.

The main element that differentiates bad carbs from good carbs is how fast the carbohydrate foods are converted into sugar in the intestine and absorbed into the bloodstream. This is known as the *glycemic index*. Foods with a high glycemic index are considered to be the bad carbs. They include white flour and white rice, refined, highly-processed flour (white breads, cereals, spaghetti, macaroni, bagels, muffins, croissants, pastries, pretzels, pancakes, waffles); fruit juices and sugar-laden sodas and sports drinks; cakes, pies, ice cream, cookies, candy, and most non-fruit desserts; chips and crackers; some vegetables, for example corn and white potatoes; sorbets, sherberts and ice cream.

The high glycemic carbohydrate foods, or the bad carbs, rapidly convert carbohydrates into glucose in the intestine, and then rapidly absorb them into the bloodstream. This rapid increase in blood sugar causes a rapid increase in the levels of insulin produced by the gland known as the pancreas. Blood glucose levels then rapidly decrease, due to the output of insulin, which results in the body's tissues and brain being actually starved for energy.

The brain then sends out hunger signals for another quick-fix meal to replenish its glucose stores. Then the rapidly fluctuating glucose and insulin levels lead to excessive calories being consumed, which have no place to go except to be stored in your body's fat cells. This invariably leads to excessive weight gain.

The increased insulin levels that are needed to fill the muscle and fat cells with sugar also inhibit the production of a muscle protein called *glucagon,* which is a protein that normally signals the body's fat cells to burn stored fuel when the blood glucose levels fall below a critical level. Since this production of glucagon is inhibited, the fat cells store more fat instead of burning fat for the production of energy. Result: Less energy produced, more fat stored. Certainly, not a pretty picture.

In addition to gaining unwanted pounds, eating foods with a high glycemic index can cause or contribute to health problems. When excess insulin is repeatedly produced by the pancreas by ingesting high-glycemic foods, the pancreas's insulin-producing cells can actually wear out, and then they begin to produce less and less insulin. This can eventually lead to diabetes.

Also, overweight and physically inactive people may develop a condition known as insulin resistance. This is a condition wherein the body's tissues resist insulin's signal to transfer glucose from the blood into the cells. This is another way that people on high glycemic diets can develop a condition known as insulin-resistant diabetes. Exercise and weight reduction are certainly ways that this condition can be prevented.

High Sugar Diets Increase Breast Cancer Risk

It appears, according to recent research reported in The Journal of Cancer Epidemiology, Biomarkers & Prevention (August 2004), that women who ate a lot of refined carbohydrates had twice the risk of developing breast cancer than those women who ate less sugars and starches. Scientists think that the excess of refined carbohydrates in the diet may increase breast cancer risk by rapidly causing the blood sugar to rise, which in turn causes a surge in blood insulin levels. These high blood insulin levels can cause normal cells to divide too quickly and may cause higher levels of insulin in the actual breasts' cells. These two factors could possibly lead to the formation of cancer cells in the breast.

These studies don't suggest that people should go on the typical low-carbohydrate diet, which essentially increases the fat (meat, cheese, and whole-fat dairy products), in their diets. These studies, however, indicate that people should restrict refined carbohydrates and substitute complex high-fiber carbohydrates in their diets. High fiber diets have been shown in many studies to decrease the risks of various types of cancer when combined with a low-fat, lean-protein diet. High-fat diets, on the other hand, have been repeatedly shown to increase the risk of various forms of cancer, particularly breast cancer. These findings raise concerns about women who eat excess amounts of refined sugars and could be at risk for developing breast cancer. This is particularly true for women who are overweight or are diabetic or who have a condition known as insulin resistance.

TIP # 4
LOSE WEIGHT WITH GOOD CARBS

According to a new Harvard study of approximately 75,000 women, participants in the study who ate at least two servings daily of high-fiber whole grain breads and cereals were fifty percent less likely to gain weight, compared to those women in the study group who ate refined carbohydrates (bad carbs) without fiber. It was shown that the high fiber good carbs burn more calories during digestion and make you feel fuller earlier and longer than eating refined bad carbs. High fiber breads, cereals, pastas and rice all reduce the output of fat-storing insulin, which results in less weight gained, and more fat calories burned. Here's yet another example of how eating good carbs can help you lose weight.

Most vegetables (except corn and white potatoes), fruits (not fruit juices), beans, legumes, nuts, whole-grain cereals and breads have a low glycemic index. These can be considered the good carbs. Your body converts these good carbohydrate foods into glucose, which is slowly processed in the intestinal tract and absorbed into the bloodstream.

Since this glucose is absorbed gradually, it only triggers a moderate, sustained rise in the insulin produced by the pancreas. This even level of blood insulin can process the blood sugar (glucose) into the body's cells slowly to use for energy production. In other words, there is no rapid filling of the fat cells full of extra sugar caused by the high levels of insulin and glucose, which causes excessive weight gain. Also, there are no rapid shifts in high or low levels of glucose or insulin, causing excess hunger and binge carbohydrate eating.

These good carbs can be helpful in a weight reduction program, provided they are combined with low-fat, low-calorie foods. These good carbs are primarily of plant origin and contain many different phyto (plant) –nutrients. They are also rich in fiber, vitamins, minerals, enzymes, and many other plant nutrients.

The following carbohydrate foods have a low glycemic index, and for all intents and purposes can be labeled as good carbs:

1.   Most vegetables, with the exception of corn and white potatoes.

2.   Most fruits with the skin intact, with the exception of fruit juices, which contain high levels of sugar and very little actual fruit. Some fruits, for example, watermelon and grapes, do have high sugar content and have to be consumed in moderation.

3.   Beans and legumes are excellent sources of fiber, protein, vitamins, minerals, and nutrients.

4.   Whole grains.

a.   Whole-grain cereals, such as oatmeal (instant oatmeals may have a high sugar content) or cold cereals are good choices for low glycemic carbohydrates. Make sure that the package shows a fiber count of, at least, 4 to 5 grams of fiber, or more, per serving, and a sugar count lower than 10 to 12 grams of sugar per serving, preferably under 8 grams. Whole-grain cereals that contain bran are usually high in fiber.

b.   Whole-grain breads. The label on whole-grain breads should show that the first ingredient listed is "whole grain flour" (example: whole-grain wheat). If it doesn't list whole-grain flour first, then it is really not a whole-grain bread. This includes any type of whole-grain bread products, especially those that also contain bran.

    c.   Brown long-grain rice makes a good low glycemic addition to any meal, since it is broken down and absorbed slowly.

    d.   Whole-wheat pastas now come in many varieties, such as noodles, spaghetti, vermicelli, linguini, etc.

5.   Nuts are good low glycemic snack foods. In addition to being absorbed slowly, they are excellent sources of protein, fiber, magnesium, copper, folic acid, potassium, and vitamin D. Nuts are also considered to be "the good fats," which are actually called monosaturated fats. They help to keep the blood vessels open, which, in turn, can reduce the risk of heart disease and strokes. Raw nuts, in particular, are called "heart healthy" nuts, since they contain generous amounts of omega-3 fatty acids. These omega-3 fatty acids are heart protective, and have also been known to prevent certain forms of cancer.

TIP # 5
LOW CARBS: HIGH PROFITS & HIGH RISK!

"Low-carbohydrate diet promoters, who make a lot of money play-ing on the ignorance of Americans, know as much about nutrition as an Arkansas hog knows about astronomy." (Carbs Are the Culprit in Popu-lar Diet Books; Family Medical Practice, October 1, 2003, p. 22.)

Most popular diet authors, including real doctors and other paramedical personnel who pretend to be doctors, know as much about nutrition as your local mechanic. Their ideas about losing weight on a low-carbohydrate diet are completely erroneous, but since most people know little or nothing about nutrition, they fall prey to all sorts of diet scams. People pay good money for pills that are supposed to burn fat from your abdomen. They buy diet shakes that contain as much fat and calories as bacon, eggs, and home fries with toast, juice, and coffee. People also believe that grapefruit juice or cabbage soup burns fat. And now people are buying low-carb beers, ice cream, and sandwiches, which are about as healthy for you as eating a hot fudge sundae, which actually has better nutrition than these low-carb foods, and actually tastes much bet-ter.

Your diet should not be restricted in any one-food source if you want to lose weight safely. A healthy diet should consist of ap-proximately 60% complex carbohydrates, 25% protein, and 15% fat. Remember that each gram of protein and carbohydrates contains 4 calories, whereas each gram of fat contains 9 calories. You do the math!

By increasing the protein content and decreasing the fat con-tent of your meals, you can slowly and safely lose weight that will stay permanently lost. Unlike with low-carb, high-profit diet scams, you won't experience rapid rebound weight gain that invariably oc-curs when you stop the diet, and you'll avoid the nasty side effects and hidden health problems inherent in these unsafe low-carb diets.

Here is the basic physiological fact that all of your low-carbohydrate diets miss: no matter what type of low-carb diet that you are currently following, it is most probably a high-fat diet. When you eat a low-carb, high-fat diet, all of the excess fat calories that you eat are stored in fat cells and end up staying there indefinitely. So the more fat that you eat, the more fat your body retains. This occurs no matter how much you restrict your carbs. Actually, the more you limit your carb intake, the more fat you will consume. These diets are filled with fat, fat and more fat that not only fills your face, abdomen, thighs, and buttocks with fat, but also clogs up your arteries with cholesterol.

However, when you consume complex carbohydrates (these are the good carbohydrates with a low glycemic index), your body expends 2 ½ times more energy converting dietary complex carbohydrates from your intestines into your bloodstream for immediate use, and then into glycogen storage in your muscles and liver, than it takes to convert fat into a source of fuel for energy production.

In other words, this means that a high complex-carbohydrate, low-fat diet causes your body to work harder after each meal, burning calories for energy, than does a high-fat, low-carbohydrate diet. This means that your basal metabolic rate (the rate at which your body operates all of its functions) is considerably higher on a high complex-carbohydrate, low-fat diet. This actually results in a higher basal metabolic rate, which, in turn, results in an additional burning of approximately 250 calories daily by the simple thermic effect of converting carbohydrates into energy.

So low-carbohydrate, high-fat diets are extremely high in saturated fats (bad fats), and, in general are unsafe and unhealthy. Low-fat diets, however, combined with complex carbohydrates (fruits, vegetables, whole-grain breads and cereals) in the diet, are healthy, safe and effective diets, and result in fast, permanent weight-loss, with no hazardous side effects.

The Partnership for Essential Nutrition cautions that low-carbohydrate diets can actually starve the brain of carbohydrates, which results in reduced energy levels and causes difficulty in concentrating. These low-carbohydrate diets can also increase the risk of kidney and liver disorders, diabetes, heart disease, stroke, gout and several forms of cancer. Many other health organizations have recently issued reports to dispel the misconceptions about low carbohydrate diets and to warn about the risks involved in their long-term use. These low-carb diets conflict with decades of proven scientific research that encourages the reduction of saturated fat and the increase of fruits, vegetables and whole grains in our diets. There is virtually no scientific basis for the simplistic belief that individuals can lose weight safely and permanently by reducing one food group (carbohydrates) from their diets. Unfortunately, the high profits garnered by the promoters of low-carb diets have resulted in significant health risks for the actual dieters.

TIP # 6
IT'S THE CALORIES, NOT THE CARBS!

The markets and the media have been flooded with low-carb food products. These food products are springing up in everything from low-carb breads and cakes to low-carb beers and marshmallows. The problem with low-carb diets is that people are just eating too many calories, most of which came from the excess fat in these unhealthy diets. Remember, that for each gram of fat you consume, you are piling up 9 calories compared with only 4 calories contained in a gram of carbohydrate or a gram of protein. It's the total number of calories that you eat daily, plus the total number of calories that you burn daily through exercise, that will make you thin or fat.

The National Academy of Science's Institute of Medicine's 2002 report on Healthy Eating recommended adults consume 45-65% of their calories from carbohydrates. This amounts to approximately 520 calories of carbohydrate daily, based on a 1,200 calorie diet.

Carbohydrates are broken down into glucose, a simple sugar that is the body and brain's preferred source of fuel. If you severely restrict the carbohydrates, then the stored carbohydrates in your muscles and liver get depleted also, and your body has to make glucose out of protein, which is an inefficient way to produce energy. This can lead to fatigue, depression, mineral imbalances, and protein loss from your body. As we have previously seen, these imbalances put a strain on the kidneys, liver, and other internal organs, and can cause damage to these organs if this type of diet is left unchecked.

The body needs carbohydrates to function properly; however, what it doesn't need is excess calories in the form of refined sugars, starches, and saturated fats. So, if you limit refined sugars, starches, and fatty foods, you will naturally cut calories from your diet and lose weight in a healthy fashion. What low-carbohydrate diets don't realize is that your body needs complex carbohydrates (whole grains, fruits, and vegetables) to function properly. These complex carbohydrates (whole-grain foods, fruits, and vegetables) are packed with nutrients and have far fewer calories than refined grains and sugar foods. These nutritionally empty carbs are not only packed with sugar, but also contain considerable amounts of fat. So, if you are eating cookies, pastries, cakes, ice cream, and the like, you are getting 4 calories for each gram of carbohydrate they contain and 9 calories for each gram of fat they contain, and if you are eating lots of meat on these ridiculous low-carb diets, then you are getting 4 calories for each gram of protein and 9 calories for each gram of fat contained in the meat. That equals a lot of extra calories in a food that really is bad for you to start with.

So, the formula is easy. Cut back on sugar and fat calories. Limit portion sizes. Eat one half now and one half later. Share food with a friend in restaurants because of the large portion sizes they serve. And most importantly, walk every day. Remember, for permanent weight-loss, you have to decrease your total calorie intake and increase your physical activity. This is really the only way to lose weight permanently and to boost energy and stay healthy.

TIP # 7
THE NET CARB SCAM

Net-carbs, or non-impact carbs, are a marketing scam to mislead the public. It is deceptive advertising. They claim that the net-carbs of a food product are the number of carbs contained in that particular food, minus the carbs from artificial sweeteners and fiber. These marketeers, or rather racketeers, claim that these carbs that they are subtracting "don't count" as carbs because they do not cause spikes in blood sugar that cause an increase in your appetite.

For instance, a popular brand of cake lists the total grams of net-carbs as 8 grams on the ingredients label; however, when you turn the box over and read the nutritional facts label, you will see that the total grams of carbs are actually 20 grams. Where did the other 12 grams of carbs disappear to? The label states that 4 grams are fiber and 8 grams are sugar alcohol. The fiber, they say, is deducted because it mostly goes through the intestinal tract without absorption. That's true, however, only for insoluble fiber. What about the soluble fiber? Where does that disappear to? It doesn't!

They also say that sugar alcohol has a minimal impact on your blood sugar, and therefore shouldn't be considered as a true carbohydrate. Sugar alcohol is neither a sugar nor alcohol. It's a bulking and sweetening agent used to add texture and taste to the food. It still is a carbohydrate, and, as such, turns to glucose in your bloodstream. It only takes a small increase in the level of blood insulin to keep the fat cells from releasing their fat. It, therefore, is the total amount of carbohydrates contained in the food, not "net-carbs," that determines the body's ability to burn fats or store carbs as fats.

There have been no studies that prove that low net-carb foods help people lose weight. Also, the Food and Drug Administration doesn't regulate using the term "net-carbs" on labels, nor does it check the different carbs that they subtract to arrive at their magical net-carb value.

The bottom line is really the total number of calories that you consume daily, which is an accurate measure of weight-loss or weight gain. Counting carbs, whether they are real carbs or net-carbs, has nothing whatsoever to do with losing real weight or maintaining weight-loss. As we have seen in the previous tips about low-carb diets being unsafe and insane, weight-loss from a low-carb diet is primarily water loss initially, followed by the unhealthy burning of fatty acids and protein. This weight that is secondarily lost is weight-loss accomplished by the unhealthy process known as ketosis. This weight-loss cannot continue indefinitely without your becoming ill. Once these dangerous low-carb diets are discontinued, then rebound weight gain comes back on your abdomen, buttocks, hips, and thighs.

So forget about counting carbs or worrying about net-carbs when you shop for foods. Concentrate on healthy foods that are low in calories and low in fat. Choose foods that contain lean protein, with moderate amounts of fiber in the form of complex carbohydrates. Concentrate on net calories lost from your diet, not bogus net-carbs on food labels.

II.
FIBER TIPS

TIP # 8
FIBER FACTS

Fiber is the general term for those parts of plant food that we are unable to digest; however, bacteria present in the colon partly digests fiber through a process known as fermentation. Fiber is not found in foods of animal origin (meats and dairy products).

TYPES OF FIBER:

Plant foods contain a mixture of different types of fibers. These fibers can be divided into soluble or insoluble, depending on their solubility in water.

1.   **Insoluble fibers** (cellulose, hemicelluloses, and lignin) make up the structural parts of the cell walls of plants. These fibers absorb many times their own weight in water, creating a soft bulk to the stool, and hasten the passage of waste products out of the body. These insoluble fibers promote bowel regularity and aid in the prevention and treatment of some forms of constipation, hemorrhoids, and diverticulitis. These fibers also may decrease the risk of colon cancer by diluting potentially harmful substances that are present in the colon.

2.   **Soluble fibers** (gums, pectins, and mucilages) are found within the plant cells. These fibers form a gel, which slows both stomach emptying and absorption of simple sugars from the intestines. This process helps to regulate blood sugar levels, which is particularly helpful in diabetic patients and is helpful in controlling weight in non-diabetics. Many soluble fibers can also assist in lowering blood cholesterol by binding with bile acids and cholesterol and eliminating the cholesterol through the intestinal tract before the cholesterol can be absorbed into the blood stream. Weight control is aided by the slower emptying of the stomach when you ingest soluble fibers. This causes a feeling of fullness and a decrease in hunger,

causing fewer calories to be consumed. For example, if you eat an apple, which has a high fiber content, you'll have a feeling of fullness, as compared to eating a cupcake, which has no fiber, and which is the same weight and size as the apple. In fact, it would take approximately three cupcakes to satisfy your brain's hunger center before you realized that you were full. Well, by then you would already have consumed 480 calories and 16.5 grams of fat. The best sources of soluble fiber are fruits and vegetables, oat bran, barley, dried peas and beans, flax seed, and psyllium.

3.   **Resistant starch**: Approximately 15% of the starch in foods is tightly bound to fiber and resists the normal digestive processes. Bacteria normally present in the colon ferment this resistant starch and change it into short-chain fatty acids, which are important to normal bowel health and may also help to protect the colon from cancer-causing agents. Foods that contain resistant starch include breads, cereals, pasta, rice, potatoes, and legumes.

4.   **Dietary fiber** is a new measurement and refers to all fiber components of plants, including crude fiber. It is, therefore, a more accurate measurement of the fiber content of foods. The dietary fiber content consequently has a higher numerical reading than grams of crude fiber. Fiber, commonly known as **bulk** or **roughage**, is the part of plant foods that cannot be digested completely, so that it passes through the digestive tract intact. Therefore, dietary fiber is the fiber content of food, which is resistant to the human digestive enzymes.

The function of fiber: The most important function of dietary fiber is to **bind water** in the intestine, in the form of a gel. This gel prevents its over-absorption from the large intestine and ensures that the stool content of the large bowel is both bulky and soft, and, consequently, its passage through the intestine is not delayed. Another important function of fiber is its effect on the metabolism, absorption, and reabsorption of **bile acids and cholesterol**. Dietary fiber actually binds or attaches to both cholesterol and bile acid, and consequently decreases their absorption from the bowel. It is now recognized that there are a number of diseases which are, at least in part, caused by a lack of dietary fiber. This was first described in 1975 by Burkitt, P.D., and Trowell, H.C., eds. in *Refined Carbohydrate Foods and Disease*, New York (London). These diet-related diseases can be classified as follows:

1. **Gastrointestinal disorders:** Constipation, diverticulosis, appendicitis, hiatal hernia, hemorrhoids, cancer of the colon.

2. **Metabolic disorders:** Obesity, diabetes, gallstones.

3. **Cardiovascular disorders:** Arteriosclerosis (coronary artery disease), varicose veins, high blood pressure and strokes.

4. **Degenerative disorders:** Breast and prostate cancer, and neurological disorders including Alzheimer's disease.

A recent study has shown that these diseases are now becoming prevalent in non-European communities, which have introduced Western dietary customs. There is almost an inverse relationship between the amount of **fiber** consumed and the prevalence of the various diseases in different countries. The higher the intake of dietary fiber, the lower the incidence of the above named disorders.

****

The latest medical report on high fiber foods indicates that there are cancer-protecting substances called phyto-nutrients actually contained in some dark green and dark yellow vegetables and fruits. One substance, known as **beta-carotene** (a nutrient that the body converts into vitamin A), is found in high concentration in spinach, carrots, broccoli, Brussels sprouts, cauliflower, winter squash, cabbage, oranges, grapefruit, apricots, and peaches. These high-fiber foods also contain large amounts of vitamin C. Both vitamins may possibly be protective against cancer of the lung, esophagus, stomach, large bowel, and skin.

TIP # 9
HOW FIBER HELPS YOU LOSE WEIGHT

1.   Fiber helps in weight-loss and weight control by the simple fact that high-fiber foods contain fewer calories for their volume. Fiber-rich foods, such as fruits and vegetables, whole-grain cereals and breads, yams and sweet potatoes, and legumes are low in fat calories and have a high water content. You are, therefore, eating less and enjoying it more.

2.   High-fiber foods have a high bulk ratio, which satisfies the hunger center more quickly than low-fiber foods; consequently, fewer calories are consumed. Fiber-rich foods take longer to chew and to digest than fiber-depleted foods, which, in turn, give your stomach time to feel full. Feeling full earlier leads to consuming fewer calories.

3.   Foods with a low-fiber content are, in most cases, considerably more concentrated in calories. These fiber-deficient foods (fats, refined sugars, flour, and alcohol) require hardly any chewing and have little or no bulk content. Therefore, large amounts of calories are consumed when eating these foods before your appetite center in the brain (appestat) is satisfied. These low-fiber foods are more concentrated in calories, so that more food must be eaten before the stomach can be filled.

4.   Removing fiber from food, such as refining grains or flours (white bread, white rice, pasta, cereal), or by extracting the juices out of whole fruits (example: apple juice, grapefruit juice, or cranberry juice) and vegetables (vegetable juices), results in the following negative features:

    a.   High-fiber foods turned into low-fiber foods.

    b.   Low-calorie foods turned into high-calorie foods.

c.   High-bulk foods turned into low-bulk foods.

d.   Longer eating time changes into shorter
        eating time, which consumes more calories.

e.   Easily satisfied hunger changes into hunger not easily
        satisfied.

f.   Complex carbohydrates slowly absorbed change into
        simple sugars, which are quickly absorbed.

g.   Slow absorption of food causes less insulin to be pro-
        duced, which changes into increased insulin production
        with subsequent weight gain.

A high-fiber diet is essentially a healthy, low-fat diet, which decreases the intake of refined and processed food. This encourages the consumption of fresh fruits, vegetables, and whole-grain cereals and breads. Fiber produces its most beneficial effect when it is eaten with each meal of the day.

Dietary fiber takes longer to chew and eat, with the subsequent development of more saliva and a larger bulk swallow with each mouthful. The larger bulk helps to fill the stomach and causes a decrease in hunger before more calories can be consumed. High-fiber diets help to provide bulk without energy and may reduce the amount of energy absorbed from the food that is eaten. These high-fiber diets are often referred to as having a low-energy density and appear to prevent excessive caloric (energy) intake. Countries that consume high-fiber diets rarely have obesity problems.

TIP # 10
FIBER-UP YOUR DIET!

1.   Drink 6-8 glasses of water daily. Fiber can absorb many times its own weight of water, providing bulk to the diet and a subsequent feeling of fullness.

2.   Eat high-fiber, whole-grain cereals for breakfast, preferably those with 5 or more grams of fiber per serving. You can beef up the fiber content of cereals by adding 1 ½ tablespoons of unprocessed bran or wheat germ, if necessary.

3.   Eat fresh fruit with skin, rather than fruit juices, which have little or no fiber content.

4.   Use whole-grain or fiber-enriched breads, which have more than double the fiber content of white bread.

5.   Consume more vegetables, legumes, and salads (without the dressing, of course, unless you use a little olive oil and vinegar). Include carrots, celery, cabbage, peas, broccoli, Brussels sprouts, lentils, potatoes with skins, dried beans, and baked beans (without sugar or bacon).

6.   Snack foods should include dried fruits, nuts, seeds, high-fiber, low-fat (1.5 grams total fat or less) snack bars, popcorn, celery and carrot sticks.

7.   Add bran, nuts, seeds, or grits to soups, yogurt, or casseroles.

8.   Use whole-grain flour or soy flour instead of refined white flour. Eat whole-grain pastas in place of regular pasta.

9.   Use whole-grain products (bran and whole-grain cereals, brown long-grain rice, and whole-grain noodles).

10.   Substitute whole-grain bread (stone-ground or whole wheat) or fiber-enriched bread and bran instead of white refined breads.

11.   Add garden vegetables (carrots, celery, cabbage, green beans, lettuce, onions, corn, peas, tomatoes, spinach, etc.).

12.   Increase fruits (apples, oranges, pears, bananas, strawberries, blueberries, plums, peaches, and cherries).

13.   Legumes, seeds, nuts, and beans are useful additions to a high-fiber diet.

14.   Unprocessed bran and wheat germ are dry bran/wheat powders, which are convenient, high dietary fibers. Each level teaspoon contains 2 grams of dietary fiber. Either may be sprinkled on cereal or other foods, or may be mixed in with orange or tomato juice to improve its taste.

15.   Breads must have the word "whole" as the first listed ingredient on the package; otherwise, it's not a true whole-grain product, no matter how the bread is labeled.

16.   Popcorn is an excellent high-fiber, low-fat, low-calorie snack. Use non- or low-fat varieties.

Start adding fiber slowly to your diet to avoid cramping, bloating, or gas. Make small additions of fiber-rich foods over a period of four to six weeks. If you find that a particular high-fiber food causes cramping or bloating, discontinue eating it and try another type of high-fiber food. Continue to increase your daily fiber intake until you reach between 25-30 grams of fiber a day for good health and weight reduction.

Remember, it's very important to drink more fluids as you increase your fiber intake. You should drink between 6-8 glasses of water daily. Fiber can absorb many times its own weight. This provides excess bulk to the diet, which makes you feel full so that you cut down on the total number of calories that you consume daily. This excess bulk formed by fiber and water also helps to keep your intestinal tract healthy.

TIP # 11
COLORFUL FRUITS & VEGGIES:
NOT JUST PRETTY FACES

It is well documented that colorful fruits and vegetables contain cancer-fighting substances and offer a full spectrum of disease prevention. For maximum health benefits, you should eat a variety of vegetables and fruits of different colors (plant pigments). The reason for the different colors is that each colored fruit or vegetable has a different phyto-chemical (phyto means plant).

These phyto-chemicals in the fruits and vegetables tend to decrease the risk of certain types of cancer. It is important to eat at least 4-5 servings of fruits or vegetables per day. The following is a list of some of the phyto-chemicals present in fruits and vegetables that can reduce your risk of cancer and heart disease:

1. Lycopene
    Lycopene is what gives many fruits and vegetables, including tomatoes, their deep red color. Lycopene is a carotenoid, or plant pigment, in the same family as beta-carotene. However, lycopene is not just a colorful addition to the fruit. Lycopene has powerful antioxidant properties that have been shown to fight different forms of cancer. National studies have shown that fruits and vegetables that contain lycopene, particularly tomatoes, may help to prevent prostate cancer, as well as colon, stomach, lung, esophageal, and pancreatic cancers, according to the American Institute for Cancer Research. Lycopene has also been linked with a lower risk of heart attacks secondary to coronary artery disease.

2. Beta-carotene
    Beta-carotene is a powerful antioxidant, which has cancer-fighting properties. For example, sweet potatoes, which are

high in dietary fiber, are loaded with cancer-fighting antioxidants (beta-carotene) and vitamins C and E. Other sources of beta-carotene are dark green, leafy vegetables, such as spinach, kale, bok choy, and other greens. Orange and deep yellow fruits and vegetables also have considerable amounts of beta-carotene, for example: pumpkins, winter squash, carrots, and cantaloupe.

3.   Flavonoids
Flavonoids are a group of phyto-chemicals found in many fruits, vegetables, and grains. The type of flavonoid that is found in grapes is called resveratrol. This compound is found primarily in the skin of grapes. It is also present in grape juice and red wine. Several studies have shown that this type of flavonoid has been instrumental in fighting cancer of the colon, liver, and breast. Resveratrol inhibits the growth of cancer by preventing the start of DNA damage in a cell and the transformation of a normal cell into a cancerous cell. It also helps to inhibit the growth and spread of tumor cells. Resveratrol also seems to be cardioprotective, according to recent medical research.

4.   Ellagic acid
This phyto-chemical is present in many types of fruits, vegetables, and grains. It appears to reduce the damage to DNA caused by carcinogens, such as tobacco smoke and air pollution. Berries contain high amounts of ellagic acid, and it has been shown that as little as a cup of raspberries or blueberries slowed the growth of abnormal colon cells in humans, and, in some cases, prevented or destroyed the development of cells that were infected with the human papillomavirus (HPV), which is the cause of cervical cancer. This particular cancer-fighting agent has also been demonstrated to have similar effects on the cancer cells of the breast and pancreas.

5.   Combinations of Antioxidants and Vitamins
Various berries, including strawberries, raspberries, and blueberries, are packed with major antioxidants, carotenoids, and vita-

min C. These antioxidants are believed to counteract the formation of many chemical processes that contribute to the formation of cancer.

6. Allium Family

Certain plants contain compounds known as allyl sulfides, which are instrumental in activating enzymes in the body that break down certain cancer-causing substances. These cancer-fighting agents increase the body's ability to excrete the cancer-causing agents. Examples of the allium family include garlic, onions, shallots, and leeks. There are many studies that have shown that people who eat lots of garlic have less cancer of the stomach and colon. It is thought that garlic blocks the growth of new cancer cells.

7. Cruciferous Vegetables

These vegetables are four-petaled flowers, which resemble crosses. Vegetables in this group include broccoli, cabbage, and cauliflower. These cruciferous vegetables, particularly broccoli, appear to protect the body against many types of cancer. Many studies have shown that people who eat an abundance of cruciferous vegetables have a reduced incidence of many types of cancer, including cancer of the colon, bladder, prostate, esophagus, lung, breast, cervix, and larynx.

8. Anthocyanins

These are plant pigments that help to protect you from heart disease. They are present in cherries, purple grapes and purple grape juice, raspberries, and strawberries.

9. Carotenoids

These compounds are antioxidant plant pigments that are converted to vitamin A by the body. There are several types: Beta-carotene is a major source of vitamin A, which lowers the risk for heart disease and certain types of cancer; lutein and zeaxanthin are carotenoids that are linked to a reduced risk of age-related macular degeneration, a major cause of blindness in older individuals.

Important sources of beta-carotene include apricots, cantaloupe, mangoes, papayas, carrots, sweet potatoes, and dark green, leafy vegetables. Important sources of lutein and zeaxanthin are green beans, greens (collard, kale, mustard, turnip), romaine and other dark lettuces, seaweed, spinach, and squash (winter types and butternut).

10.   Isoflavones
These compounds act as weak estrogens (phytoestrogens). Eating approximately 100 milligrams of isoflavones daily can improve bone density. Good sources of isoflavones are soy milk, soy protein, tofu, and textured vegetable proteins.

11.   Indoles
Indoles are compounds that help to fight cancer. Good examples of foods with indoles are broccoli, Brussels sprouts, cabbage, and cauliflower.

12.   Folic Acid
This B vitamin helps prevent birth defects and lowers levels of homocysteine, which is an amino acid linked to heart disease. Excellent sources of folic acid include oranges, broccoli, romaine and other dark lettuces, and spinach.

So, you can see that fiber is not just another pretty face. It is a face of multiple colors, wherein each fruit and vegetable has its own individual face derived from its own plant pigments. Each one of these colorful fruits and vegetables offers a full spectrum of disease prevention.

TIP # 12
FOODS THAT BLOCK FATS AND BURN CALORIES

Dietary fiber is one of your best foods to block both the absorption of fat and to burn up extra calories. Sounds almost too good to be true; however, it really works.

First of all, when you combine the high-fiber foods that we have already discussed (see list of high-fiber foods), combined with any fat in your diet, like a piece of cake or a hamburger, each gram of fiber traps fat globules by entwining them in a fiber-like web, made up of thousands of fiber strands. Once these fat globules are trapped in the fiber's web, they pass through the intestinal tract before they are absorbed into the bloodstream. Therefore, these fat globules are excreted in the waste material from your colon without getting absorbed and stored as fat in your body. The fiber is actually removing the fat from your body like a garbage truck removes garbage. And to underscore that fact, fat really is garbage.

Secondly, fiber actually burns up calories by itself. This is accomplished because fiber causes your intestinal tract to work harder in order to digest the fiber foods. The body's metabolism therefore uses more energy for this time-consuming digestion, and as a result can actually consume most of the calories that the fiber foods contain. Strange as it seems, some heavily fibered foods can actually burn up more calories than the fiber foods contain, thereby creating a deficit of calories. This causes the body to use stored body fat for the production of energy. Each gram of fiber that you consume can burn up approximately 9 calories, most of which come from fat. So if you eat 30 grams of fiber a day, you can actually burn up an additional 270 calories daily (30 grams fiber x 9 calories). You can actually subtract those 270 calories every day from your total daily calorie intake, without actually cutting those calories from your diet.

In addition to blocking fat and burning calories, fiber foods bind with water in the intestinal tract and form bulk that makes you feel full early in the course of your meal. So you eat less, and therefore you consume fewer calories at each meal. Also, your appestat (hunger mechanism) is satisfied for longer periods of time, since it takes longer to digest fiber foods, and therefore you will have less of a tendency to snack between meals.

TIP # 13
FIBER: LOSE WEIGHT & STAY HEALTHY!

New findings from The Nurses' Health Study in 1998/1999 show that fiber, especially cereal products, protects against heart disease. This study examined the relationship between fiber consumption, as reported by nearly 70,000 women from 1984 through 1998. Woman who ate an average of 23 grams of fiber a day had a 47% lower risk of major coronary events, including myocardial infarction and/or fatal coronary heart disease, compared to those who ate about half as much fiber. When the researchers analyzed the individual effects of three different fiber sources (fruits, vegetables, and cereals), only cereal fiber significantly reduced the risk of cardiovascular disease.

A daily bowl of cold whole-grain breakfast cereal that supplies 5 or more grams of fiber cut heart disease risk by approximately 37%. This study was reported in the Journal of the American Medical Association in 1999. In this particular study of 70,000 women by The Nurses' Health Study, the ages of the women ranged from 37 to 64 years of age. None of the women in the study had a previous diagnosis of heart disease, stroke, cancer, diabetes, or high cholesterol. It is proposed that the increased consumption of whole-grain products may increase insulin sensitivity and lower triglyceride levels. Also, whole-grain products, including cereals, are important sources of phytoestrogens and may favorably affect blood coagulation activity (JAMA, October 27, 1999, volume 282, number 16).

Fiber Reduces Risk of Strokes

The nutrients in fruits and vegetables, such as dietary fiber and antioxidants, are associated with a lower risk of heart disease, but few studies have examined their relationship to the risk for stroke. This study, reported in the Journal of the American Medical Association, described the association between fruit and vegetable intake and ischemic stroke in over 70,000 woman enrolled in The Nurses' Health Study and 38,000 men in the health professional follow-up study. Everyone in this particular study had no history of cardiovascular disease, stroke, cancer, diabetes, or high cholesterol.

During the follow-up period, which included fourteen years for women and eight years for men, each increment of one serving of fruit or vegetables per day was associated with a 7% reduction for risk of ischemic stroke in women and men. This would translate into a *35% reduction in stroke for people* who ate five servings daily of fruit and vegetables. This study showed that there was no further reduction in the risk of stroke above 5-6 servings of fruit and vegetables per day. The consumption of a variety of vegetables and fruits, such as cruciferous vegetables (examples: broccoli and cabbage), green, leafy vegetables, citrus fruits or vitamin C-rich fruits and vegetables resulted in the largest decrease in risk. These are pretty impressive results for sticking to your high-fiber diet of fruits and veggies (JAMA, October 6, 1999, volume 282, number 13).

Fiber K.O.'s Heart Disease

In a recent study in the American Journal of Clinical Nutrition, women who ate three to four servings of whole grains a day had one-third to one-half the risk of developing heart disease as opposed to women who ate refined flour, such as white bread. It is important to check the ingredients in any commercial food to see that it is truly made from whole grains. In particular, it is important to check the ingredients in snack foods (for example, cookies, crackers, and chips), since many of these products contain not only refined white flour, but also partially hydrogenated oils (trans-fats), which actually can raise our cholesterol more than any other types of saturated fats.

In a recent study in the American Journal of Epidemiology, people on a high-fiber diet showed a significantly reduced risk from coronary heart disease and death from all causes. This study reviewed dietary data from the Scottish Heart Study on approximately 12,000 women and men, 40-59 years of age. Women with a high intake of fiber had the greatest reduced risk of mortality from all causes, including coronary heart disease. These results suggest that the current public health drive to increase your fiber intake to at least five portions of fruit and vegetables a day should have beneficial effects on all causes of mortality.

These researchers attributed the beneficial effects of fiber to the fact that folate, the antioxidant-active flavonoids, and minerals (selenium, magnesium, and copper) will be co-ingested at higher levels in high-fiber, fruit and vegetable rich diets. In addition, the stool-bulking properties of fiber may play an important role in maintaing good health. Along with fiber, the study participants ingested other nutrients present in fruits and vegetables that may have an added effect on the prevention of coronary heart disease and on all types of mortality.

Reduce Risk of Alzheimer's Disease

A recent Harvard Medical School study found that middle-aged people who regularly ate cruciferous and leafy green vegetables, delayed the onset of the mental decline that normally comes with aging. Middle-aged people who were overweight had twice the risk of later developing dementia, according to a study at the 9th International Conference on Alzheimer's disease. Eating lots of vegetables, and staying physically and socially active may significantly reduce the risk of developing Alzheimer's disease according to several other recent studies.

TIP # 14
FEARLESS FIBER

Soybeans: The New Fiber Health Food

Soybeans contain soy proteins, which help to reduce the risk of cardiovascular disease. The reason for this is that soy proteins reduce the amount of total fat LDL cholesterol in the blood by affecting the synthesis and metabolism of cholesterol in the liver. Its amino acid composition differs from the structure of other proteins found in meat and milk.

Clinical trials showed a significantly lower incidence of coronary heart disease in patients with a high soy intake. Soybeans can be found in many different varieties, including soy beverages, tofu, tempeh, soy-based meat substitutes, and some baked goods. However, to qualify, such soy-rich foods should contain at least 6.5 grams of soy protein and less than 3 grams of total fat per serving, with less than 1 gram of saturated fat per serving, to qualify as a heart-healthy food. One-half cup of cooked soybeans contains 4 grams of fiber.

In another related study, soy supplements were shown to cut the risk of developing colon cancer in half. Soy supplements also decreased the relative risk of having a recurrence of colon cancer in high-risk subjects. This study was reported at the annual conference of The American Institute for Cancer Research. High soy intake may be able to delay the onset of colon cancer in those at risk, or may lead to more cancer-free years in those whose initial cancer was surgically removed.

Soy foods, vegetables and fruits contain isoflavinoids, which can offset some of the adverse effects of estrogen on the body. Also, by eliminating meat from the diet, the levels of estrogen in the body decrease. By decreasing meat and increasing fiber, the body is less likely to develop estrogen-related uterine and breast tumors.

Veggies Decrease Risk of Bladder Cancer

In a recent study on bladder cancer, it was shown that in order to reduce the risk of bladder cancer, it is necessary to drink lots of fluids, not to smoke, and to eat lots of cruciferous vegetables. A high intake of cruciferous vegetables, particularly broccoli and cabbage, significantly reduced the risk of bladder cancer. This may be explained by the presence of one or more phyto-chemicals in broccoli and cabbage, which are specific in the reduction of bladder cancer risk. This study also showed that a high intake of fruits, yellow vegetables, and green, leafy vegetables did not significantly reduce the risk of bladder cancer. The relationship with high cruciferous vegetable intake (broccoli and cabbage) was associated with the highest reduction in the risk of developing bladder cancer.

Veggies Help Prevent Breast and Uterine Cancer

Women who limit their intake of red meat and eat lots of green vegetables have a reduced risk of developing breast cancer and uterine cancer. High levels of estrogen, which results from the consumption of beef, ham, pork, and other red meat, have been implicated in the formation of breast and uterine cancer. The intake of 4-5 servings of fruits and vegetables daily containing phytonutrients, in particular, isoflavinoids, may offset some of estrogen's effect on the uterus and breast (Obstetrics and Gynecology, 94 [No.3]: 395-398, 1999).

Fiber and Fibroids

Benign uterine fibroids are the most commonly diagnosed uterine tumors. They have been associated with anemia, pelvic pain, and, in some cases, fertility problems. It appears that women who have high levels of estrogen, which may be related to red meat intake, are more prone to fibroids. A recent study showed that diets decreasing or eliminating meats and increasing green vegetables have a significant effect on the prevention of the development of fibroids.

The vegetables and fruits contain isoflavinoids, which can offset the effect of estrogen on the body. Also, by eliminating meat from the diet, the levels of estrogen in the body decrease. By decreasing meat and increasing fiber, the body is less likely to develop estrogen-related uterine fibroid tumors.

Fiber and Colon Cancer

In January 1999, a group of Boston researchers reported no difference in the rates of colon or rectal cancer in women who ate a high-fiber diet, as opposed to those who ate a low-fiber diet. This study was eventually refuted by qualified researchers who pointed out that, in this particular study, the only type of fiber that was studied was exclusively cereal fiber.

Women, for example, metabolize fiber differently from men. Female hormones also helped protect against colon cancer in many cases, as they do against heart disease. Moreover, with so many different kinds of fiber included in a healthy diet, the evidence of scientific studies on the impact of plant foods and their fiber is still in its infancy.

Recent studies have subsequently shown that high fiber diets, which include not only cereal grains, but also fruits and vegetables, do, indeed, help to prevent the development of colon cancer. As part of the ongoing Nurses' Health Study that provided the data questioning the preventive role of fiber, a 2002 report showed that women who ate a diet high in red meat had higher rates of colorectal cancer.

In that same study, both men and women whose diets were low in red meat and high in fruits, vegetables, and cereal grains had a significantly decreased risk of colon cancer. In countries where diets are high in plant-based foods and low in red meat and animal fat, people have lower rates of heart disease and colon cancer.

TIP # 15
TOP 20 ANTIOXIDANT FOODS

Fruits	Veggies	Honorable Mention
Apples	Broccoli	Apricots
Blueberries	Bok choy	Cantaloupe
Blackberries	Cabbage	Cauliflower
Cherries	Carrots	Greens (others)
Cranberries	Garlic	Mangoes
Prunes	Kale	Nuts
Purple grapes	Spinach	Olive oil
Raisins	Squash	Oranges
Raspberries	Sweet potatoes	Tea
Strawberries	Tomatoes	Whole grains

Blueberries May Reverse Aging Process

New research has indicated that women on antioxidant-rich diets showed fewer age-related disorders than those on a normal diet. The studies showed that among all the fruits and vegetables, the benefits were greatest with blueberries, which reversed age-related effects, for example, loss of balance and lack of coordination. They also discovered that blueberry extract had the greatest effect on reversing aging decline. Antioxidants help neutralize free radical byproducts on the conversion of oxygen into energy, which, if not neutralized, can cause oxidative stress and lead to cell damage.

Previous studies have shown that both strawberries and spinach extract can also help to prevent the onset of age-related defects. However, the greatest effect was shown in patients who ate blueberries. Phytonutrients in blueberries, particularly flavonoids and beta-carotene, seem to have an anti-inflammatory effect, which may even help in the prevention of Alzheimer's disease. Again, we have another solid recommendation for eating fruits and vegetables because of their high fiber content and because of their phytonutrient and antioxidant powers (The Journal of Neuroscience, September 15, 1999; 19: 8114-8121).

Spinach: The Health Powerhouse

If you're looking for a vegetable with super healing powers, try spinach. It's packed with vitamins, antioxidants, and minerals that will protect you from many diseases. Spinach contains many antioxidants, including beta and alpha carotenes, lutein, zeaxanthin, potassium, magnesium, vitamin K, and folic acid. Recent studies at two major universities have found that, as strange as it seems, eating spinach may lower your risk of strokes, colon cancer, cataracts, heart disease, osteoporosis, hip fractures, memory loss, Alzheimer's disease, depression, and even birth defects. The disease-fighting properties in spinach are better absorbed when spinach is cooked with a little olive oil. Now, that's what I call a super, super vegetable.

Oranges Protect Your Heart and Fight Cancer

In a recent study, it was shown that oranges boost the good HDL cholesterol, in addition to providing vitamin C, folic acid, and numerous flavonoids. These compounds are thought to prevent cholesterol oxidation, which has been linked to a reduced risk of coronary events.

An orange or two a day will keep atherosclerosis away. Researchers have found that citrus fruits, in particular oranges, also showed anti-cancer activity in animals and in test tubes. These researchers found that animals that ate oranges for several months were 25% less likely to develop early colon cancer than animals given only water. Compounds such as liminoids in oranges seem to alter the characteristics of the colon lining, discouraging cancer growth. These researchers speculate that oranges may also help to suppress breast cancer, prostate, and lung cancer.

Protecting Your Eyesight With Veggies

Kale and spinach are two vegetables rich in the antioxidants *lutein* and *zeaxanthin*. These antioxidants have been reported to protect against age-related cataracts and macular degeneration, one of the leading causes of blindness. Also high in these vision-protecting antioxidants are romaine lettuce, broccoli, collards, turnip greens, and corn.

Broccoli: Beats the Big Three

Scientists have known for years that eating certain leafy green vegetables can cut your risk of developing certain forms of cancer. A new medical study, however, has shown that eating broccoli and broccoli sprouts may also reduce your risk of heart disease, high blood pressure, and stroke. Broccoli and broccoli sprouts have high concentrations of the antioxidant *glucoraphanin*, which has been shown to boost the body's defense mechanism against cancer-forming free radicals.

A recent study reported by the University of Saskatchewan reported that laboratory animals who were prone to high blood pressure and were fed broccoli sprouts with high levels of glucoraphanin, had lower blood pressure, less inflammation, a stronger immune system, and less incidence of heart disease and strokes. Newer studies have reported similar findings in humans, who consumed abundant amounts of these leafy, bushy, dark green vegetables.

The following **10 antioxidant foods** have been shown to have extremely high anti-cancer activity:

1. Soy beans
2. Ginger
3. Licorice
4. Celery
5. Cilantro
6. Parsley
7. Parsnips
8. Onions
9. Brussels sprouts
10. Mushrooms

TIP # 16
SNACKS THAT KEEP WEIGHT OFF

High fiber snacks that keep your weight off and satisfy your appetite include raw vegetables and fruits; whole-grained crackers, breads and cereals; soups with lots of vegetables and 100% vegetable juices; nuts and dried fruits; and popcorn among others. These high fiber snacks combine with water in your intestinal tract and form what's known as "bulk," which satisfies your hunger mechanism quickly. This combination of fiber and water takes longer to digest, and therefore your appetite stays satisfied for a longer period of time. This bulk fills you up without filling you out. Stay away from snack foods that contain refined carbohydrates like cookies, pretzels, crackers, and candies. These refined sugars increase rather than decrease your appetite by spiking both blood sugar and insulin levels. And besides, these refined carbohydrates help to store unwanted fat in your abdomen, buttocks and thighs.

For snacks that satisfy your appetite for a long period of time, without raising your blood sugar and insulin levels, choose from a wide array of high fiber snack foods. For example, soups (not creamed) with lots of veggies make an excellent mid-day snack for appetite control. Several companies have come out with new travel-type containers for soup that can be eaten on the go, with or without heating-just like drinking a can of soda. Also, 100% vegetable juices come in plastic travel bottles, which make an excellent high fiber, appetite-satisfying snack, that's also chock-full of essential nutrients, vitamins and minerals.

Cut-up fruits and veggies, packed in sealed plastic baggies make excellent high fiber, nutritious, appetite satisfying snacks that you can take with you anywhere. Dried fruits such as figs, prunes and apricots also are great travel snacks that are high in fiber, low in calories and fats and high in essential nutrients, vitamins and minerals. These fruit and veggie travel packs are appetite satisfying and loaded with nutrients like B-complex vitamins, potassium, folic acid, magnesium and iron among others.

To keep your weight off and boost your energy level, combine your high fiber snacks with lean protein. Try peanut butter with or without low sugar jelly or low fat cheese on whole-wheat crackers, bread or pita. Be especially careful that you stay away from packaged snacks like peanut butter crackers, which are loaded with the very bad trans fats. You can even add wheat germ or instant oatmeal to low fat yogurt or cottage cheese for a delicious fiber-protein snack. Sliced low fat turkey or low fat cheese on one slice of whole wheat bread or English muffin, makes a stick to your ribs, long-lasting snack.

When you combine high fiber foods with protein, your body's metabolism processes this fiber-protein complex much more slowly than it would by eating either fiber or protein separately. Subsequently, the digestion and absorption of this fiber-protein complex takes place at a slower rate, which results in less calories consumed because your appetite is satisfied more quickly and for a longer period of time. It takes the body considerably longer to digest and absorb protein than it does for the body to process carbohydrates and fats. Protein causes a very gradual rise in the blood sugar, which, in turn, causes a very moderate rise in insulin levels. Therefore, the addition of lean protein to your high fiber snack ensures that you'll be hunger-free until the next meal, without the desire for additional snacking.

Nuts alone or combined with a small box of raisins, makes a great high quality fiber-protein snack mix, to help keep your weight off. Nuts are high in protein, fiber and essential nutrients such as folic acid, potassium, magnesium, selenium and healthy monounsaturated fatty acids. Nuts, particularly walnuts and almonds, have been shown in numerous studies to help prevent heart disease. A one-ounce serving of nuts either alone or combined with a small box of raisins, is an excellent way to boost your energy level and satisfy your appetite for many hours.

Popcorn is a great high fiber, low calorie, low fat snack that's easy to make anywhere. The hot-air popcorn-popper ensures a virtually fat-free, high fiber snack; however, the non or low fat microwaveable varieties are also great, as long as you check to see that the butter or fat content is not too high. Popcorn can be mixed with peanuts, raisins, apple slices and other fruits for variety. You can even bake your popcorn with cinnamon, peanut butter, raisins, fruit, Parmesan cheese and even garlic.

A plastic baggie of your favorite dry high fiber, whole grain cereal, makes an excellent transportable nutritious snack to take with you anywhere. The addition of some dried fruit to your travel cereal pack can add flavor and nutrition to your weight control snack. Even the varieties of cereals that are lightly sweetened are great diet snacks provided they're high fiber, whole grain, low sugar and low fat cereals. Check the ingredients label to make sure that there are no more than 1.5 grams of total fat and no more than 8 grams of sugar. Also make sure the cereal has at least 5 grams or more of dietary fiber. There's no need to check the amount of carbohydrates in the cereal, since as we've seen in the section on carbs, counting carbs is bogus. It has nothing whatsoever to do with weight-loss.

TIP # 17
HIGH FIBER FOODS

FRUIT GROUP: Each serving of the below-named fruits has approximately 2 grams of fiber.

1 apple or pear	1½ oz. box raisins
1 banana	1 medium peach
½ cup of strawberries	2 small plums
1 small orange	10 large cherries

BREAD GROUP: Each serving has approximately 2 grams of fiber.

Whole-wheat bread	Bran muffin (low fat)
Wheat bread (cracked)	Stone-ground bread

CEREAL GROUP: Each serving has approximately 2 grams of fiber.

Shredded wheat–½ biscuit	Oatmeal–½ cup
Puffed wheat–1 1/3 cups	Wheat bran–½ cup
Corn flakes–2/3 cup	Grape Nuts–½ cup

Cereals highest in fiber are 40% Bran, All-Bran, Grape Nuts, Fiber One, Shredded Wheat, Whole Wheat Flakes, Raisin Bran, Multigrain Cheerios, and Multigrain Chex. Check the ingredients label and look for 5 or more grams of dietary fiber on the label.

VEGETABLE GROUP: Each serving has approximately 2 grams of fiber.

1 cup celery	2 cups lettuce
1 corn on the cob	½ cup green beans
½ cup baked beans	1 medium potato
1 medium raw tomato	4 Brussels sprouts
1 stalk of broccoli	1/3 cup carrots

The following vegetables are highest in fiber: artichokes, green beans, cabbage, cauliflower, Brussels sprouts, dried beans, lima beans, and peas.

MISCELLANEOUS GROUP: Each serving has approximately 1 gram of fiber.

2 ½ tsp. peanut butter	10 peanuts
3 tsp. strawberry jam	1 large pickle
1 cup popcorn	2 tsp. relish

TIP # 18
COUNT FIBER, NOT CARBS!

High-fiber foods, such as fruits, vegetables and whole grain products, generally require a longer time to eat, since they require more chewing and give your brain's appetite center time to shut down early. Also, when fiber foods are combined with water in the intestinal tract, they become bulky and create a feeling of fullness, which again prevents you from overeating. However, when you eat low fiber foods, more food is ingested before a sense of fullness has been attained. Low fiber refined carbohydrate foods are usually eaten more quickly, and since they require less chewing and are not bulky, they enter the intestinal tract more rapidly, where they are quickly absorbed as sugars. This rapid rise in blood sugar causes a spike in insulin production, which stores more fat in the body and then quickly drops the blood sugar, which in turn makes you hungry again. Therefore, since it takes a certain amount of time for nerve impulses to reach the appetite control center, the feeling of hunger is not shut off until excessive amounts of low fiber refined carbohydrates are eaten. This is the primary reason that low fiber foods invariably cause weight gain.

SPINACH AND DARK GREEN LEAFY VEGETABLES

These greens are low in calories and are filling because of their fiber content and their crunch factor. Crunchy fiber foods take longer to eat and help your brain's hunger mechanism to shut down quickly. Fiber also helps to prevent the absorption of fat from the intestinal tract by wrapping threads of fiber around the fat globules, thus preventing the fat's absorption into the blood and actually sweeping the fat through and out of the intestinal tract before it is absorbed.

Green leafy vegetables also contain many plant nutrients, antioxidants, and B-complex vitamins, which help to prevent cancer, heart disease, and degenerative neurological diseases.

OATMEAL

Fiber-rich oatmeal is nutritious, tastes great, and is slow to digest. The high insoluble fiber content of oatmeal causes your appetite mechanism to shut down early because of its slow rate of absorption from the intestinal tract. Oatmeal has also been shown to reduce your craving for high-refined sugar products and fatty foods.

Oatmeal is also high in soluble fiber, which helps to clean out the fat in your blood vessels by increasing the HDL cholesterol, which sweeps out the bad LDL cholesterol from the bloodstream. Oatmeal for breakfast every day has been recommended by the American Heart Association as a great start for your day to reduce your risk of heart disease.

People who eat oatmeal, as well as other whole-grain bran-type cereals daily, have less than one-half the risk of developing obesity and diabetes as non-cereal eaters. High-fiber bran cereals help to regulate insulin production in the morning. This helps to control your appetite and reduce the risk of gaining unwanted pounds.

Bran cereals are also packed with magnesium, which is a mineral that can also reduce your risk of developing diabetes. Magnesium also helps to stabilize your blood sugar by preventing the overproduction of insulin by the pancreas. Oatmeal and whole-grain bran-type cereals are a great way to start your diet every morning.

TOMATOES

Tomatoes are unique in their ability to produce an amino acid called *carnitine*. This amino acid causes your body to burn fat at a faster rate by increasing your body's basal metabolic rate. Any tomato products, from ketchup to tomato sauce, are great for your weight-reducing diet.

Tomatoes also contain abundant amounts of vitamin C and an antioxidant called *lycopene*, which helps to prevent several types of cancer, including breast and prostate cancers. The combination of vitamin C and lycopene also helps to prevent the buildup of cholesterol in your bloodstream.

BEANS

The high fiber content of beans helps to reduce the absorption of both fat and calories from the intestinal tract. The fiber content of beans reduces your appetite and lets you eat fewer calories because you get filled up earlier.

Beans are also high in potassium and low in sodium, which helps to reduce the risk of high blood pressure and strokes. Beans, beans – they're good for the heart, the more you eat them, the more you're smart.

SWEET POTATOES

Contrary to popular belief, sweet potatoes are excellent sources of vitamins and minerals and are considered good carbs. They are a great addition to any weight-loss program because of their high fiber content and their nutritional value.

Sweet potatoes are good sources of vitamin C, B-complex, folic acid, potassium, vitamin A, and beta-carotene. These nutrients, combined with plant sterols found in sweet potatoes, are powerful antioxidants, which can help to lower cholesterol and lower your risk of heart disease. When sweet potatoes are eaten with their skin, they are good sources of both insoluble and soluble fiber. These two types of fibers help to reduce your appetite the way most fiber foods do, by filling you up and satisfying your appetite early, without supplying extra calories in your diet.

ASPARAGUS

Asparagus is an excellent source of potassium, folic acid, beta-carotene, vitamin C, and the antioxidant *glutathione*, which helps to fight nasty free radicals, which can damage normal cells. Asparagus is a great addition to any diet program, since it is low in calories and high in fiber and nutrients.

Steamed asparagus is great eaten alone or in a salad. It must be refrigerated or frozen quickly to prevent the loss of its nutritional value. If boiled too long, most of the nutrients end up in the water.

PEPPERS

Red and green and yellow sweet peppers are excellent sources of vitamin C, vitamin A, and beta-carotene, B-complex vitamins, potassium, and folic acid. Since they are low in calories and high in fiber, peppers are excellent foods to add to your weight-loss program. Due to the spices contained in peppers, they have a tendency to satisfy your taste buds early and aid in reducing your appetite.

Peppers contain antioxidants that help to prevent blood clots by decreasing the blood platelet's stickiness. This property can help to prevent heart attacks and strokes. Hot peppers contain higher quantities of antioxidants than sweet peppers. They also contain phyto-nutrients that help to prevent certain forms of cancer. Hot peppers also contain an ingredient called *capsaicin*, which makes these peppers hot and spicy. This ingredient has anti-inflammatory properties and helps to relieve the pain of various forms of arthritis and nerve inflammations. These capsaicinoids can cause eye irritation if transferred from your hands to your eyes, so be careful to wash your hands thoroughly after handling hot peppers.

III.
NEW DIET TIPS

TIP # 19
WHAT DO THE FRENCH PEOPLE KNOW?

The French Paradox

There are three known factors contributing to atherosclerosis (hardening of the arteries):

1. Overactive platelet activity, which causes blood to stick and can lead to a heart attack or stroke.

2. High levels of LDL (bad) cholesterol. Free radicals can oxidize LDL cholesterol and contribute to the buildup of plaque in the arteries.

3. The third contributing factor to atherosclerosis is damage to endothelial cells.

Patients on a diet high in purple grapes had an almost tripling of the blood vessels' ability to respond to the increased blood flow, and also showed a slower onset of LDL oxidation, meaning that it is less likely that the oxidation will contribute to atherosclerosis. The flavonoid (transresveratrol) in purple grapes is the key to the prevention of atherosclerosis. Fruits, vegetables, nuts, and seeds also contain flavonoids, as well as red wine. This research is often referred to as the French Paradox, which helps to explain the low incidence of heart disease in France, where red wine consumption is high.

While people in France eat almost three times as much saturated fat as Americans, the French have only one-third the risk of heart disease. The same heart disease prevention benefits appear to be related to the consumption of purple grapes, which contain the same flavonoids as red wine (Circulation, October 1999, 100: 1050-1055), which increases the good HDL cholesterol.

Eating purple grapes or grape juice gives similar protection against heart disease without the alcohol content. Both purple grapes and grape juice contain the flavonoid, transresveratrol, which have cardio-protective benefits. The International Journal of Cancer (Nov. 2004), has found that the antioxidant resveratrol, also appears to have a protective effect against prostate cancer.

The French also eat three to four more servings of vegetables daily than Americans eat. Also, the French season their vegetables with heart-friendly olive oil and add herbs, nuts, and spices. They also take time in preparing their food, and relax and eat slowly to enjoy their meals. Americans, on the other hand, usually eat fast foods or prepare meals quickly and eat them just as fast. They don't savor foods like the French people do and consequently don't take the same care in the food preparation and presentation.

Whatever the reasons are, the French people have only had an 8-10% rise in obesity over the last decade compared to a 20-25% increase in obesity in the American population. Also, the French have considerably less heart disease and breast cancer compared to Americans. French people rarely eat prepackaged foods, which are filled with saturated fats, sugar, and sodium. They also usually sauté or grill their fresh vegetables to bring out the natural sugars and nutrients contained in the vegetables.

The portions of meats that they eat are relatively small in comparison to the amount of fresh vegetables that they consume. And even though they enjoy desserts with a high fat content, they usually only consume small portions of these tasty morsels. So, it is not only the wine that keeps the French people healthy, it's their preparation and enjoyment of healthy, fresh foods, and their relaxed manner of eating slow, leisurely meals. The French take time preparing and eating their meals, unlike their American counterparts who eat quickly and often have little knowledge of what they've actually eaten. Perhaps, it's the Americans' quick, stressful lifestyle and their inability to relax that causes heart disease and not the actual diet at all.

TIP # 20
A MEDITERRANEAN DIET FOR YOU!

Research shows that the Mediterranean Diet, which emphasizes whole grains, greens, fruits, vegetables, and olive oil, is healthier then the typical American diet, which is high in fat and processed foods. There is a significantly decreased risk of heart disease and cancer in the Mediterranean cultures, which have been thriving on these foods for thousands of years.

The Mediterranean Diet can be explained quite simply by explaining what whole grain actually is. Grains consist of three layers: 1) the inner germ, 2) the middle endosperm, and 3) the outer bran. Processing white flour and white rice keeps the two inside layers, but removes the outside layer, the bran, with its fiber, vitamins, and minerals. With whole grains, you get all of those nutrients plus complex carbohydrates, protein, fiber, antioxidants, and phytochemicals, which may help guard against cancer and heart disease.

Also, whole grains provide energy and calories with little fat, and then lengthen the time that it takes to digest foods, so that you feel full longer. This simple explanation of why the Mediterranean Diet is far superior to our Western diet shows us why fiber is a significantly important factor in weight reduction and good health. Weight control is aided by the slower emptying of the stomach when you ingest soluble fibers. This causes a feeling of fullness and a decrease in hunger, causing fewer calories to be consumed.

The Mediterranean Diet is rich in olive oil, vegetables, legumes, fish, chicken, fruits, and pasta, with infrequent consumption of red meat. This diet was associated with approximately a 35% reduction in the risk of mortality due to coronary heart disease and a 25% reduction in the death rate due to cancer. It appears that eating the Mediterranean Diet is associated with significantly reducing inflammatory proteins that are present in our bloodstream. One marker in particular, called the C-reactive protein, has been associated with an increased risk of heart disease. It appears that the Mediterranean Diet lowers this C-reactive protein, thus decreasing the risk of heart disease.

Mediterranean people have a significantly lower risk of heart disease and cancer than Americans have. Most of their benefit is provided by their liberal use of olive oil. Although their diets contain 25-35% fat calories, this fat is monounsaturated, heart-healthy fat. Mediterraneans use olive oil and olives in almost everything they eat. It is used in pastas, breads, vegetables, salads, fish, and even in cakes and pastries, which are cooked with olive oil. Also, the Mediterranean people eat less animal fat than most countries, including the United States, and consume significantly more fruits, vegetables, and whole grains.

Olive oil's monounsaturated fats help to increase the good HDL cholesterol and decrease the bad LDL cholesterol. This leads to less cholesterol blocking your arteries and a significantly lower incidence of heart attacks and strokes. Olive oil also contains certain antioxidants called polyphenols, which have cancer-protective qualities.

And if all that isn't enough to help the Mediterranean people keep healthy, they also have a secret weapon that most Americans know or care little about. Walking! Mediterraneans, in addition to eating healthy, walk almost all of the time. They walk to work, to visit friends, or just to leisurely stroll through their cities and countrysides. They climb up and down hills and keep in good shape with little or no thought to their aerobic activity. Walking just comes naturally!

In two separate studies reported in the September, 2004 issue of the Journal of the American Medical Association, it was reported that the mortality rates were 65% lower in elderly people who followed the Mediterranean Diet combined with 30 minutes of daily walking. The Mediterranean Diet consisted primarily of olive oil rather than butter or margarine, legumes, nuts, seeds, whole grains, vegetables, potatoes, fruits and fish. These people also consumed very little meat and whole fat dairy products.

Researchers found that people on the Mediterranean Diet had a significant decrease in body weight, blood pressure, cholesterol and triglycerides, and blood sugar and insulin levels. These individuals also had a significant increase in the good HDL cholesterol, which helps to prevent heart disease. This 12-year study followed approximately 2,500 men and women ages 70-90 in 11 different European countries.

In a separate study it was reported that the Mediterranean Diet helped people lose weight by changing the body chemistry, by reducing dangerous insulin abnormalities and chronic inflammation of arteries and other tissues in the body. This diet reduced the incidence of the *metabolic syndrome*, which causes the accumulation of fat around the abdomen and increases the risk of diabetes, heart disease, cancer and Alzheimer's disease.

TIP # 21
SUPER FAT-BURNING FOODS

New research suggests that drinking two glasses of skim milk or eating two cups of yogurt or one serving of cheese per day may produce weight-loss with no actual reduction of the calories in your diet. It appears that the mineral calcium burns stored fat, while promoting the buildup of more muscle tissue. This unique combination of calcium and protein, which is present in milk, yogurt, and cheese, helps the body to burn fat and store protein. Remember, nonfat milk and low-fat cheeses, and nonfat or low-fat yogurts have the same minerals, vitamins, protein, and calcium as whole milk without the added fat content.

Several new studies have shown that people who regularly drink skim milk and eat yogurt lose an average of 1½ pounds per month, with no change whatsoever in their diets. It is believed that calcium decreases the stores of fat in the fat cells by actually burning stored fat. Also, it is thought that the protein present in milk, yogurt, and cheese replaces the fat stored in the fat cells by its unique process of providing extra protein to the body's cells. This protein is used by the body's cells as the natural building blocks to activate all of the body's cells, tissues, and organs' metabolic functions. A recent study at the University of Tennessee suggests that the calcium found in these foods actually blocks fat storage in the cells that plump up your abdomen, thighs, and hips. Another similar study reported in Quebec showed that taking at least 1,000 milligrams of calcium per day increases the good (HDL) cholesterol and decreases the bad (LDL) cholesterol. And as far as your diet is concerned, fat-free milk contains 220 milligrams of calcium and only 80 calories per glass.

What better snack food than a glass of skim milk could you find, that lowers your cholesterol and reduces your waist size at the same time? When you combine these new findings with lowering the total fat intake in your diet, which naturally cuts calories, and by adding a moderate exercise program, you have the ideal weight reduction, fat-burning tip. Other high-calcium and fat-burning foods include cheese, tofu, nonfat cottage cheese, spinach and collard greens, and calcium-fortified fruit juices; however, be careful of the high sugar content in fruit juices.

SOY PRODUCTS (Soy milk, soy yogurt, tofu, etc.)

Soy contains natural phyto-nutrients called isoflavones. These plant chemicals break down the fat, which is stored in your body's fat cells. Several studies have confirmed that the consumption of soy products on a regular basis helps dieters burn fat and lose weight without any other alteration in their diets.

These isoflavones present in soy also have been shown to reduce the incidence of heart disease. In addition to helping you lose weight by breaking down the stored fat in your body, isoflavones also break down saturated fat in your blood, thus lowering the LDL bad cholesterol. Soy products are good for the heart and great for your figure.

LOW OR NONFAT DAIRY PRODUCTS (Milk, cheese, and yogurt)

The calcium present in these low-fat milk products has been shown to block the absorption of fat from the intestinal tract. Less fat absorbed, less fat stored. Simple! New medical research has proven that people who ate at least one serving of a low or nonfat milk product daily lost considerably more weight than those dieters who ate no calcium-containing dairy products.

The calcium present in these low or nonfat dairy products has also been shown to reduce the risk of heart attacks and strokes by increasing the HDL good cholesterol in the blood and by reducing the stickiness of the blood platelets, which can cause blood clots.

Low-fat dairy products have also been shown to rev up your metabolism, thus causing your muscles to burn more fat. By increasing this fat-burning effect, you get less fat stored in your fat cells and you will lose more weight gradually, which stays lost permanently.

TIP # 22
KEEP THE WEIGHT OFF

A new study presented at the North American Association for the Study of Obesity in November 2004, showed that low-fat diet plans work better at keeping weight off compared to low-carbohydrate diets. This particular study used The National Weight Control Registry that evaluated more than 2,500 people from 1995 to 2003, ages 40 to 50, in an effort to learn the secrets of success from those people who had lost 30 pounds or more and kept them off for at least one year. Physicians compared their diets to see if one type of diet or another made any difference in how much weight they lost and how much weight they regained one year later.

The type of diet (low-fat or low-carb) made no difference in how much weight people lost initially. In fact many of the dieters had lost an average of 50-60 pounds initially. However, those individuals on the low-carbohydrate diet who subsequently increased their fat intake over the next year regained the most weight. These low-carb dieters ate fewer carbohydrates while keeping the amount of protein in their diets the same. Instead of replacing carbohydrates with more protein, these low-carb dieters replaced the carbohydrates with additional fat in their diets. This increase in dietary fat resulted in the low carb dieters regaining almost all of the weight that they had originally lost.

Similar studies have also shown that low-carb dieters eventually regain all or most of the weight that they have originally lost. More than one half of Americans who have tried low-carb diets have given up, according to a recent survey. The American Institute for Cancer Research used these trends to issue a statement in September 2004 urging dieters "to come back to common sense" and to eat a balanced diet by increasing fruits, vegetables, and whole grains, reducing portion size, and increasing physical activity.

In two related studies presented at the November, 2004 meeting of the North American Association for the Study of Obesity, it was shown that walking was an effective method for losing and maintaining weight loss.

This particular study showed that walking was an excellent alternative for individuals who hate to exercise. Walkers tend to continue their walking programs compared to people who work out at a gym and often give up strenuous exercises, either because of boredom, injury or time constraints.

In one study, 180 overweight people followed a 40-week weight-loss program. These individuals limited their calorie intake to 1,200 to 1,500 calories per day. They participated in one of three exercise programs. Two groups either worked out for 45 minutes in a gym or at home four days per week. The third group walked an average of two miles per day. At the end of 20 weeks all three groups lost similar amounts of weight, approximately 7-8% of body weight. At the end of 40 weeks they had lost approximately 8-9% of body weight. After 2 years most of the exercisers had regained some of their weight with the exception of the walkers who managed to maintain most of their initial weight-loss. Walkers seem to be able to continue a long- term exercise program quite easily, as opposed to those people trying to fit time-consuming strenuous workouts into their busy schedules.

In another related study presented at this conference, women who ate between 1,200 to 1,500 calories per day and followed one of three exercise plans, lost an average of 22 to 28 pounds in six months. The exercise plans consisted of a walking program alone, a walking and yoga program and finally a walking and strength-training exercise plan. There was no significant difference in the amount of weight lost or weight maintained in any of the three groups. Strength training or yoga can be important components in a fitness program. Strength training in particular, helps to build strong bones and muscles. However, the one consistent finding was that walking was the main factor responsible for losing weight and keeping the weight off in all three of the exercise plans. Walking is considered to be the great weight-loss equalizer.

Walking regularly every day combined with a low fat, lean protein, high fiber diet appears to be the best way to lose weight and to keep that weight off permanently. This combination of a healthy low-fat diet and walking has been shown repeatedly to be the easiest and safest method to lose weight quickly and keep the weight off, stay fit and trim, and lead a healthier longer life.

TIP # 23
FAST FOOD TIPS: THE WORST
AND THE BEST

Most fast foods are so high in calories, saturated fats, and sodium that they not only make us fatter, but they also cause the buildup of fat in our arteries, causing heart attacks, strokes, and high blood pressure.

The Worst

1.   The average double cheeseburger, with large fries and a large soda, contains approximately 1,800-2,000 calories, and approximately 100 grams of fat, of which almost 40 grams are saturated fat. It also contains approximately 1,500 mg of sodium. So, for most people, that amounts to the number of calories that they would consume in one day and three to four times the amount of fat and salt that they would consume in any given day.

2.   Two slices of pizza with extra cheese and/or meat contain 750-800 calories, 35-40 grams of fat (15 grams of saturated fat), and 2,000 mg of sodium.

3.   Fried fish sandwiches contain approximately 700 calories, 40 grams of fat (15 grams of saturated fat), and 1,200 mg of sodium.

4.   Nachos with cheese and sour cream contain 1,200-1,300 calories, 80 grams of fat (25 grams of saturated fat), and 2,500 mg of sodium.

5.   A chocolate milkshake contains almost 800 calories and 40 grams of fat, of which 25 grams are saturated.

6.   A large coke contains 200 calories.

7.   Large fries contain 600+ calories, 20 grams of fat, and 10-12 grams of saturated fat.

8.   Fried chicken or a fried chicken wrap with cheese and sauce contains 700 calories and 44 grams of fat (12 grams of saturated fat), and 2,000 mg of sodium.

The Best

1.   Choose a single hamburger without cheese or sauce. Add lettuce, tomato, and onion, with or without ketchup or nonfat mayo, and skip the fries and order a diet soda.

2.   Order a grilled chicken sandwich without the mayo, or better yet, a grilled chicken Caesar salad with fat-free herb vinaigrette dressing (on the side).

3.   A good choice is a small vegetable chili without cheese.

4.   Soft chicken taco without sauce.

5.   Pizza without extra cheese or meat; add fresh veggies to increase the nutrition content.

6.   Order a large salad plain, or add grilled chicken, and add fat-free dressing (on the side).

7.   Roast beef sandwich without the sauce.

8.   If you must have fries, order the smallest bag and either split with a friend or toss it in the trash when you are finished less than one-half of the bag.

TIP # 24
POWER FOODS BOOST NUTRITION

The 2005 Dietary Guidelines by the U.S. Department of Agriculture and the Department of Health and Human Services have included the following recommendations for improved nutrition:

1. Eat fruits, vegetables, and whole grains at each meal.
2. Limit trans-fats by avoiding processed and refined foods.
3. Avoid foods with increased amounts of sugar and salt.
4. Limit saturated fatty meats and substitute chicken and turkey without the skin and seafood.
5. Replace whole milk dairy products with low-fat or non-fat milks, cheeses, and yogurts.
6. Increase intake of monounsaturated fats such as nuts, seeds, avocados, and olive, canola and peanut oils.

There is a group of foods that I refer to as **Power Foods**, which deliver more nutrition per calorie than processed and refined foods. These foods are not only packed with vitamins but contain many different types of nutrients that are unique to these foods. These nutrients consist of plant (phyto) nutrients, flavonoids, monounsaturated fats, omega-3 fatty acids, complex carbohydrates, proteins, minerals, fiber, and a whole host of nutritional boosting compounds that are found in these nutritious power-foods. Among these unique, healthy, energy-boosting foods are the following groups:

Green Leafy Vegetables: These vegetables include spinach, romaine and other dark lettuces, kale, bok choy, chard, collard greens, and seaweed. These foods are excellent sources of beta-carotene, B complex vitamins, folic acid, and antioxidants known as carotenoids. These nutrients and antioxidants help to reduce the risk of certain eye and neurological disorders and also help to prevent heart disease and certain forms of cancer.

Cruciferous Vegetables: These four-petaled vegetables include broccoli, cabbage and cauliflower. Cruciferous vegetables are an excellent source of complex carbohydrates and dietary fiber. Several studies have shown that people who eat an abundance of cruciferous vegetables have a reduced incidence of several types of cancer. These vegetables are good sources of beta-carotene and B-complex vitamins.

Orange Vegetables: These vegetables include carrots, sweet potatoes, pumpkins, butternut squash, winter squash, and cantaloupe. These orange vegetables are loaded with cancer fighting antioxidants (beta carotene and vitamin C and E).

Tomatoes: Tomatoes are unique in their ability to produce an amino acid called carnitine, which helps the body burn fat at a faster rate by increasing the body's basil metabolic rate. Tomatoes also contain abundant amounts of vitamin C and an important antioxidant called lycopene, which helps to reduce the risk of several types of cancer. Cooking tomatoes helps to release this important antioxidant, lycopene, from the tomatoes.

Beans and Lentils: These power foods are high in fiber and are excellent sources of protein, without the fat found in meats and dairy products. The high fiber content of beans and lentils help to reduce the absorption of both saturated fat, cholesterol, and calories from the intestinal tract. The fiber content of beans and lentils reduces your appetite and may reduce the risk of heart disease. These foods are rich in potassium, iron, zinc, B6, and folic acid.

Berries and Grapes: Blueberries are packed with antioxidants and fiber and are low in sugar and calories. Blueberries have a significant effect on reversing age-related disorders due to their antioxidants which help to neutralize dangerous free radicals. Blueberries contain phytonutrients, particularly flavonoids and beta-carotene, which have an anti-inflammatory effect, which may even help to prevent the onset of Alzheimer's disease. Cranberries are also low in calories and contain vitamin C and antioxidants called procyanidins, which keep the urinary tract healthy. Strawberries and raspberries are also packed with antioxidants, carotenoids, and vitamin

C. Purple grapes contain vitamin-C, potassium, and a flavonoid called transresveratrol, which helps to reduce the risk of heart disease.

Citrus Fruits: Oranges, lemons, tangerines, and grapefruit contain antioxidants and are high in vitamin C, potassium, and folic acid. They provide the body with essential nutrients.

Nuts and Seeds: Nuts, particularly walnuts and almonds, are rich in the heart-healthy monounsaturated fats and are excellent sources of fiber and protein. Nuts are excellent sources of folic acid, vitamin D, copper, and magnesium. Seeds like flax, sunflower, and pumpkin are an excellent source of a phytoestrogen called lignans, which have a balancing effect on the body's hormones and are an excellent source of antioxidant properties. Seeds are also abundant sources of protein, iron, vitamin E, and phosphorus.

Omega-3 Fatty Acids: Seafood, in particular, salmon, trout, and tuna, are good sources of protein, nutrients, and omega-3 fatty acids. These omega-3 fatty acids may help to reduce the risk of heart disease and prevent the development of certain forms of cancer. Flax seed oil also contains omega-3 fatty acids.

Monounsaturated Fats: Olive oil, olives, canola, and peanut oil, as well as nuts and avocados, contain the heart-healthy monounsaturated fats. These fats help to reduce the bad LDL cholesterol and raise the food HDL cholesterol and can help to offset the bad effects of eating too many omega-6 fatty acids contained in processed foods that are made with the vegetable oils (corn, sunflower, cottonseed and safflower oils).

Whole Grains: Whole grain breads and cereals, especially those that contain bran, are excellent sources of fiber, B-vitamins, minerals including zinc, iron and magnesium. All whole grain foods help to reduce your appetite because of their high insoluble fiber content. Oats in particular are also high in soluble fiber, which helps to clean out the fat in your blood vessels by increasing the good HDL cholesterol, which sweeps out the bad LDL cholesterol from the bloodstream.

TIP # 25
FRUITS THAT REDUCE YOUR APPETITE

Oranges and grapefruit contain both soluble and insoluble fiber along with a particular form of fiber called **pectin**. The pectin fiber in these fruits suppresses your appetite while providing you with only 70 calories. Oranges and grapefruit also contain many plant nutrients that help to lower blood fats and strengthen your immune system. Eight ounces of orange or grapefruit juice, on the other hand, contain approximately 130-150 calories and are loaded with refined sugars, which cause your insulin levels to spike and results in sugar being metabolized into fat cells.

Apples are another natural hunger suppressant, since they contain both soluble and insoluble fiber. One medium apple with the skin contains approximately 4 grams of fiber. It also contains pectin, which, combined with the fiber, has a tendency to decrease hunger pangs after you've finished a nice big juicy apple. This decrease in hunger occurs because the soluble fiber content of the apple plus water in your digestive tract forms bulk in the intestines, which actually makes you feel full. Also, the pectin content of apples suppresses your appetite by tricking your brain's hunger center (appestat) into believing that you are full, when all you've really eaten is one delicious apple. This multi-fiber food fills you up without filling you out. The high fiber content of apples also helps to lower your blood pressure and your blood cholesterol and has been shown to decrease the incidence of colon polyps and colon cancer.

The actual chewing time of eating an apple and the slower digestion due to the formation of bulk (fiber + water) gives your appetite control mechanism time to shut down, so that you feel full earlier. By contrast, eating a piece of cake, which has no fiber and lots of sugar, never stimulates the appestat to shut down, and consequently your body doesn't know you are full before you have had time to consume two or three pieces of cake. Similarly, you can also eat a cheeseburger, French fries, and a large coke, way in advance of your brain knowing that you are full.

This is because these foods contain lots of fat and refined carbohydrates, which are absorbed quickly, and again increase the blood sugar and blood insulin levels, which leads to hunger.

Apple cider vinegar contains several acids that act as digestive enzymes. These acids (malic and tartaric acid) help to break down carbohydrates slowly, which in turn slows their absorption into the bloodstream. The tart flavor of apple cider vinegar also increases the production of saliva, which also contains enzymes that aid in slower digestion of carbohydrates. You can add 1 Tbs. of apple cider vinegar to salads for its appetite-suppressing effect. Raspberry vinaigrette dressing (nonfat) also contains some of these appetite-suppressing components. Any type of vinegar dressing, such as olive oil and vinegar, has the ability to suppress your appetite. Just remember to use these dressings in extremely small amounts, or else the calories from the oil will start to build up.

TIP # 26
CALORIES DON'T COUNT –
NOT REALLY!

According to a recent study in the Journal of the American Medical Association's April 2003 issue, there is a no magic formula to losing weight. You can lose weight by following a variety of different diet programs; however, the one thing that always counts are the number of calories that you consume vs. the number of calories that you burn daily.

Yes, even those horrendous, low-carbohydrate diets work also, but that's because they restrict calories also, not just carbohydrates. Also, they work because you are creating an unhealthy condition found in diabetics called ketosis, where you are burning protein instead of fat to lose weight. Unfortunately, the weight comes back twice as fast when you stop the diet, if, however, you are fortunate enough not to have damaged your liver or kidneys while you were on this unsafe diet.

Unfortunately, Americans have been gaining so much weight in the last twenty years that obesity is becoming an actual epidemic. Over 60% of adults are overweight, which includes approximately 30% who are considered obese. This trend has almost tripled in teenagers during this same time period.

After reviewing over one hundred diet studies since 1966, the researchers concluded that if you want to lose weight, you should consume fewer calories daily over a long period of time. By restricting one type of food over another, as in the low-carbohydrate diets or high-protein diets, you are essentially making a weight loss program more difficult, and essentially more dangerous.

A low-fat, high-fiber diet with moderate amounts of protein and complex carbohydrates is the single, best healthy weight-loss diet that you can follow for good health and permanent weight -loss. There are no dangerous side effects, no feelings of hunger, and along with permanent weight-loss, you have the added benefit of a diet that is actually good for you. You will lose weight and have a lower incidence of heart disease, hypertension, strokes and several forms of cancer. This diet, by its very nature, turns out to be a low-calorie diet in disguise, and what's more, it actually works and keeps on working. It is a diet plan that you can follow for a lifetime to lose and maintain your ideal weight, and maintain good health, longevity, and physical fitness.

TIP # 27
QUICK WEIGHT-LOSS TIPS

1. Drink one cup of fat-free milk instead of one cup of whole milk. Add nonfat milk to your coffee, cappuccino, or lattes.

2. Use 1 tablespoon of mustard, ketchup, or fat-free mayonnaise instead of regular mayonnaise in salads or on sandwiches. Mix ketchup and nonfat mayonnaise to make a delicious Russian dressing. Served on a wedge of iceberg lettuce, it makes a tasty snack.

3. Share a small bag of potato chips or French fries with a friend, or skip them altogether, or just taste three or four and throw the bag away.

4. Cut a slice of pizza in half and save the other half for later in the day.

5. Check serving sizes of your favorite foods when you eat out. For example:

    a. One-half cup of cooked cereal or pasta at home is equivalent to a single serving size; however, restaurant portions are equivalent to approximately three serving sizes, and that's before they even add the sauce.

    b. One-half of a bagel is one serving, but a deli bagel is equivalent to at least three servings.

    c. One small pancake or waffle at home is equal to one serving size, but in a restaurant, one large pancake is about two and one-half servings.

d.   A dozen potato chips or tortilla chips equals approximately one serving; however, a small bag contains at least two to three servings.

6.   Always check the serving sizes on any prepackaged food that you get. You will be surprised that some of them say that the contents contain two or three serving sizes. Most people, when they consume of package of processed foods, assume that it is one serving size, when, in actuality, it may be two to three serving sizes.

7.   Be careful of prepackaged foods that contain trans fats. Trans fats are identified as partially hydrogenated oils. They are not listed or labeled on the package as trans fats. The FDA will be requiring foods to have trans fats listed, but that won't occur until 2006. The reason trans fats are dangerous is that they raise the blood levels of cholesterol and saturated fats and lead to heart disease, hypertension, and strokes.

8.   When you order a meal in a restaurant and the serving size seems too large, tell the waiter immediately to wrap-up one half of the meal before you start to eat. Don't wait until you've started the meal to decide to take some of the food home. By that time, you'll probably have eaten more than half of the portion size and your calorie count will go sky-high. When you've finally discovered that you've had enough to eat, the usual response is: " Well, that's really not enough food to wrap-up and take home."

IV.
PROTEIN TIPS

TIP # 28
HEALTHY PROTEIN

It is important to add lean, healthy protein to your diet in the form of:
1.   Very lean meat, fish, and poultry without skin.
2.   Nonfat milk and low-fat cheeses, including yogurt.
3.   Vegetable protein, including tofu, beans, nuts, and legumes.

The addition of low-fat protein to your diet makes you feel less hungry, since it short-circuits the appetite control mechanism (appestat) in the brain. It takes your body longer to digest protein than it does to digest fat or refined carbohydrates. Protein causes a very gradual rise in the blood sugar, which, in turn, causes a very moderate rise in insulin levels and a satisfaction of hunger.

Adding healthy protein to your diet is easy. The following types of protein are considered healthy:
1.   Low-fat protein foods, including fish, lean white meat of chicken or turkey, without the skin, and very lean meats, particularly lamb and pork as opposed to beef, which has an extremely high fat content.
2.   Dairy products. Nonfat milk and low or nonfat cheeses, yogurt, egg whites, and tofu are excellent healthy proteins.
3.   Vegetable proteins. Nuts, beans, legumes, and tofu.

When you are on a low-calorie diet, your body needs more protein for the production of energy and your body's cell maintenance. We are not talking about protein in the form of cheeseburgers, hot dogs, bacon, butter, and fat, fat, and more fat, as proposed in many of the popular low-carbohydrate diets. These are considered unhealthy, high-fat proteins.

What we are suggesting is the addition of small amounts of lean protein with each meal to give the body the building blocks for your body's metabolism. Protein can help significantly to modify your hunger longer than high-fat or high refined-carbohydrate meals.

High-protein diets, which concentrate on limiting your carbs cause weight-loss initially; however, you are losing weight because you are eating fewer calories, not because you are consuming fewer carbs. So it is very important to cut back on refined sugars and starches, and substitute low-fat protein (chicken, turkey, fish, egg whites, nonfat milk and cheeses, and yogurt) in their place. Also, add lots of fresh fruits and vegetables to increase the good carbs (complex carbohydrates) to provide energy for all of your daily activities.

Also, when you reduce calories, your energy intake is compromised, so that adding more lean, nonfat protein to your diet makes some of the protein that you eat available for the production of energy. Adding lean protein to your diet satisfies your appetite quicker and longer than high-carbohydrate, high-fat foods. It takes the body considerably longer to digest and absorb protein than it does for the body to process carbohydrates and fats. This results in a gradual rise in blood sugar and only a moderate production of insulin. In other words, you avoid the roller coaster ride of high and low blood sugars, and high and low levels of insulin in the blood, causing excessive hunger.

TIP # 29
HARMFUL PROTEIN

Most high-protein diets are actually unsafe, since they are based on severely limiting your carbohydrate intake. In other words, they are low-carbohydrates in disguise. Most of these so-called high-protein diets have you eating three to four times more protein than the recommended dietary allowance, and, in most cases, the high protein that you are actually eating is the harmful, high-fat protein foods. These include fatty meats, sausage, ribs, bacon, ham, whole-milk cheeses, whole milk, and butter, oils, and eggs. These high-fat protein products contain high levels of artery-clogging saturated fat, along with their protein content. For example, a double cheeseburger has a fair amount of protein, but it also has close to 75 grams of fat, 25 grams of which are saturated fat.

High-protein diets tax your kidneys by making them work harder to flush out toxins and waste products from the body. These risks are compounded for people who have preexisting medical problems, such as diabetes, high blood pressure, heart disease, or an unknown pre-existing kidney disorder. Even if you take in excess amounts of fluids daily with these high-protein diets, it may not be sufficient to flush out these body toxins. Check with your doctor, who can order blood tests to see if you have caused your kidneys any damage on one of these high-protein diets.

These high-fat, high-protein diets can actually leach out calcium from your bones. This is caused by the protein being broken down to uric acid in the bloodstream, which, incidentally, is also harmful in excess amounts, since high levels of uric acid can cause gout and contribute to the formation of kidney stones. Your bones then release their calcium in order to neutralize the acid in the blood. Even by adding calcium supplements to the diet, you cannot replace this calcium that has been lost from the bones. If this calcium loss continues for a long period of time, the bones actually become thin and a condition known as osteoporosis results.

These harmful high-protein diets can contribute to certain forms of cancer (breast, prostate, and colon) because of the high saturated fat contained in these diets, particularly in meat. Meat, in addition to its high fat content, is also chockfull of hormones and other nasty contaminants, such as bacteria, viruses, and a newer addition known as prions. These prions are thought to be responsible for the development of mad cow disease.

It certainly is no surprise to hear that elevated blood cholesterol, heart disease, and strokes can, and often do, result from these high-protein, high-fat, artery-clogging diets. I have had many patients whose blood cholesterol levels have reached unhealthy levels on these high protein diet plans.

High-protein diets that are also high in fat can cause a condition known as ketosis. Ketosis occurs when your body breaks down fat into acetone and ketone bodies to be used as a fuel for the production of energy to be utilized by the brain. This results because the high-protein diets, which are exceptionally low in carbohydrates, remove the necessary carbohydrates that are needed to be broken down as fuel. This condition, known as ketosis, is unhealthy, because it upsets the chemical balance of the blood and can result in kidney damage.

Ketosis is the same abnormal condition that results in people with diabetes when their blood sugars are out of control. It is an abnormal metabolic condition in diabetes, as well as in people on these high-protein, low-carbohydrate, high-fat diets.

Other side effects of these unhealthy diets include bad breath, which is a tip-off that your body is in ketosis. Constipation is often a result of these high-protein, high-fat, low-carbohydrate diets, because you are limiting the amount of fiber in the form of vegetables, fruits, and whole-grain cereals and breads.

TIP # 30
TASTY PROTEIN MEALS

Balance your meals by adding a small amount of lean protein to each meal. Combine that with healthy high-fiber, complex carbohydrates and your appestat (appetite control mechanism in the brain) will feel satisfied easily, and you will be less hungry after eating a balanced meal.

If you eat refined carbohydrates, such as baked goods, white bread, white rice, white potatoes, low-fiber breads and cereals, and sugar-containing desserts, then you have refined carbohydrates that are broken down rapidly in the intestinal tract and just as rapidly absorbed into the bloodstream as sugar (glucose). This rapid rise in blood glucose causes a rapid rise in insulin and a rapid increase in your hunger.

In order to balance your meal plans, stick with complex carbohydrates that are high in fiber and low in sugar. These include fruits, vegetables, whole-grain breads and cereals, whole-grain pastas, nuts, and legumes. Balance these meal plans with small amounts of protein, including lean meats, poultry, fish, eggs, nuts, beans, and low-fat dairy products (milk, cheese, yogurt, tofu, cottage cheese, and sour cream - - all low-fat varieties).

Snack on nuts instead of cookies, which will satisfy your hunger and are considerably more nutritious than sugar snacks. Even low-fat cookies and cakes and pastries are extremely high in sugar.

TASTY PROTEIN SNACKS

1. Blend a smoothie with 1 cup of fat-free milk with the fruit of your choice (bananas, strawberries, blueberries, peaches, etc.).
2. Whole-wheat muffin or bagel (scooped out) with 1 Tbs. of low-

fat peanut butter, with or without low-sugar jelly or jam.

3. 1 slice of whole-wheat pizza with light cheese topped with veggies.

4. Carrots or celery sticks dipped in fat-free, low-calorie dressing or in salsa.

5. 2 ounces of grilled salmon or chicken, with mixed greens. Fork-dip your low-calorie dressing of choice as you enjoy this tasty snack.

6. Low-fat cheese, 2 slices, and tomato melted on a whole-wheat muffin or bagel (scoop out bagel).

7. 1 cup of low-fat cottage cheese or yogurt with the fruit of your choice.

8. Small chicken Caesar salad with Romaine lettuce, low-fat Parmesian grated cheese, 1 oz. grilled chicken breast and low-fat Ceasar dressing on the side.

9. Tuna melt with low fat cheese on 1/2 whole wheat bread or muffin with sliced tomato.

10. 2 slices of low fat turkey breast on one slice whole wheat bread with non or low-fat mayo or mustard and lettuce and tomato.

11. One ounce of mixed nuts (walnuts, almonds, peanuts) with one small box raisins.

12. Hard boiled or poached egg on one slice of whole wheat English muffin.

TIP # 31
QUICK BREAKFAST TIPS

- 1 slice cinnamon French toast with egg substitute and whole-wheat bread.

- 1 cup fat-free yogurt with fresh fruit and 1 Tbs. wheat germ.

- 1 nonfat waffle with fresh fruit topping.

- 1 toasted small whole-wheat bagel with 1 tsp. nonfat cream cheese.

- 1 cup cooked oatmeal with cinnamon and 1/4 cup raisins.

- 1 cup cold bran-type or whole-wheat cereal with 1/2 cup any fresh fruit.

- 1 poached egg with 1 slice whole-wheat toast and 1 tsp. all-fruit jam.

- 1 fried egg with nonfat spray and 1 slice whole-wheat bread and 1 tsp. all-fruit jam.

- 1 scrambled egg with nonfat spray and oat bran or whole-wheat English muffin with 1 tsp. all-fruit jelly.

- 2 egg white or egg substitute omelet with 1 slice low-fat (skim milk) cheese, tomato, onions, green peppers, mushrooms (any or all).

- A scooped-out whole-wheat bagel with 1 slice unsalted smoked salmon (nova lox) with nonfat cream cheese, tomato, and onion.

- 2 small whole-wheat or buckwheat pancakes made with egg substitute, topped with fresh fruit and/or sugar-free syrup.

- 1 fried egg with nonfat spray and two small veggie nonfat sausages or two slices nonfat turkey bacon.

TIP # 32
SLIMMING LUNCH TIPS

- 1 veggie burger on whole-wheat bread or bun with lettuce, tomato, onion, and ketchup.

- 1 Tbs. reduced-fat peanut butter and 1 Tbs. jelly sandwich on whole-wheat bread.

- 2 Tbs. nonfat cream cheese sandwich on whole-wheat bread with sprouts, tomato, cucumber, and lettuce.

- 1 nonfat cream cheese (2 Tbs.) and jelly (1 Tbs.) sandwich made with whole-wheat bread.

- 1 medium whole-wheat pita pocket with tuna (3 ounces) packed in water, with lettuce, tomato, cucumber, sprouts, and 1 tsp. Dijon mustard or 1 tsp. nonfat mayonnaise.

- 1 medium whole-wheat pita pocket with grilled chicken breast (3 ounces) and 1 tsp. nonfat mayonnaise with lettuce, tomato, celery, and cucumber.

- 1 whole-wheat sandwich with two slices skim-milk cheese (Alpine Lace) or other low-fat cheese, with lettuce, tomato, shredded carrots, and sprouts, with mustard or 1 tsp. nonfat mayonnaise.

- 1 whole-wheat bun with two slices reduced-fat turkey breast, with lettuce, tomato, mustard, or 1 tsp. nonfat mayonnaise.

- 1-cup soup (minestrone, lentil, split pea, or any vegetable or bean-based soup) with 1 small whole-wheat roll.

- 1 soft corn tortilla with 1/3-cup fat-free refried beans, with shredded low-fat cheese, lettuce, tomato, and salsa.

- 1 medium order steamed mussels or clams (12) with 1/2-cup marinara sauce with 1 small whole-wheat roll.

- Chicken Caesar salad with lettuce, tomato, chopped celery, cucumber, and with 3 ounces grilled chicken breast and non-fat Parmesan cheese and 1 Tbs. fat-free Caesar dressing.

- 1/2 veggie hoagie (tomatoes, lettuce, olives, peppers, onions, cucumbers, carrots, sprouts – your choice) with scooped-out Italian roll, leaving only shell.

- 1 whole-wheat bagel, scooped out, with 1 slice smoked salmon (nova lox) with tomato, onion, and lettuce.

- 1 whole-wheat bagel, scooped out, with 2 slices low-fat cheese, grilled with tomato and Dijon mustard or 1 tsp. non-fat mayonnaise.

- 1 can (3 ounces) sardines (drain oil) on whole-wheat bread or pita with tomato, lettuce, and onion.

- 1 slice pizza (tomato or with light cheese and tomato), topped with veggies of your choice and a side salad with 1 tsp. non-fat dressing.

- Nicoise salad with mixed greens, tuna, string beans, tomato, anchovies, 1/2 sliced hard-boiled egg, olives, radishes, celery, onions, and bell pepper with mustard vinaigrette dressing on the side (dip fork in dressing sparingly), and one scooped-out French roll.

TIP # 33
DINNER WITHOUT RECIPES

- 1 grilled 3-ounce, lean hamburger on whole-wheat roll with lettuce, tomato, onion, and ketchup, and 1 small white potato made into oven-baked French fries (slice into fries, spray nonstick pan with nonfat spray, and bake at 400° until crisp).

- 1 small can fat-free baked beans, 1 nonfat beef hot dog or turkey dog on whole-wheat bun with sauerkraut, relish, and mustard, and small side salad with 1 tsp. nonfat dressing.

- 1 small can sardines (drain oil) or tuna packed in water in large tossed salad of lettuce or romaine, tomato, cucumber, pepper, onion, sprouts, carrots, and olives, and 1 tsp. nonfat dressing or mustard vinaigrette dressing.

- 1-cup spinach fettuccine with fresh vegetables and 1/2-cup tomato or marinara sauce and large tossed salad.

- 1-cup whole-wheat spaghetti with 12 clams or mussels, garlic, 1/3 cup white wine, 1 tsp. olive oil, and seasoning, and large tossed salad.

- 3-ounce grilled salmon steak or salmon fillet with tomatoes, onions, peppers, and garlic, and small baked potato or yam with skin and 1 cup steamed vegetable (your choice).

- 1-cup Chinese greens with 6 medium grilled shrimp and garlic with 1-cup brown rice.

- 2 soft tacos with nonfat refried beans, lettuce, tomato, onion, and grated nonfat cheese, with 3 ounces sliced grilled chicken and salsa.

- 3 ounces lean roast beef with horseradish and small baked potato or yam with skin, 1 cup steamed veggies, and small whole-wheat roll.

- 6 medium cooked, peeled shrimp with cocktail sauce and small ear of corn, and 1 cup steamed asparagus, broccoli, or spinach.

- 3 ounces broiled or baked cod, halibut, mackerel, or sole with grilled onions, peppers, mushrooms, and tomatoes, with lemon, wine, and seasonings, small whole-wheat roll, and tossed salad.

- 2 small lamb chops (trim fat) with 2 tsp. mint jelly and whole broiled tomato, with 1 small baked sweet potato and tossed salad.

- Goat cheese salad with reduced-fat goat cheese, mixed greens, tomato, olives, bell peppers, cucumber, celery, with mustard vinaigrette dressing on the side (dip fork in dressing sparingly), and 1 scooped-out Italian or French roll with tomato, low-fat mozzarella cheese, basil, and lettuce.

- Spinach salad with 1 ounce low-fat blue cheese, 1/2 ounce chopped walnuts, sliced apples, cherry tomatoes, cucumbers, and 1 Tbs. dressing made with mustard, lemon, and 1 tsp. olive oil.

- 1-cup low-fat macaroni and cheese with 1-cup zucchini, diced tomatoes, onions, and garlic, and an ear of corn or a small sweet potato and steamed fresh carrots (1/2 cup).

TIP # 34
NUTS TO YOU!

Nuts to you! Actually nuts, particularly walnuts and almonds, which are rich in monounsaturated fats, cause the brain to release a hormone called *cholecystokinin*, which actually shuts down the appetite control mechanism in the brain and prevents hunger. Two ounces of almonds is enough to release this appetite-suppressing hormone. The monounsaturated fats contained in nuts also have heart-protective properties.

These monounsaturated fats can lower blood cholesterol, particularly the bad LDL cholesterol, and they can also help to reduce blood pressure. Previously thought to be high in fat, recent studies have shown both the health benefits and the weight reduction properties of nuts. Nuts are packed full of nutrition. They contain folic acid, vitamin D, copper, magnesium, fiber, and healthy monounsaturated fats.

Nuts help to prevent heart disease by retaining your blood vessels' natural elasticity, which, in turn, keeps the arteries open. This fact helps to reduce the incidence of high blood pressure and heart disease.

Nuts are also packed with protein, which is good for you and acts as a natural appetite suppressant by the very nature of its slow digestion and subsequent absorption into the bloodstream. Almost all of the energy contained in the protein you eat is burned as fuel for your body's metabolic functions; therefore, hardly any of the calories contained in dietary protein are converted into fat storage. Therefore, nuts are not only good for you, but they don't put on extra weight. And what's more, they taste good. Well, nuts to you! Always remember to limit portion size to a handful because of the extra calories contained in nuts.

Nuts contain monounsaturated fats that help to suppress your appetite so that you eat fewer calories. The benefits of eating nuts are good taste, high crunch factor, appetite-suppressing and fat-burning weight-loss benefits rolled into one, healthful, good-tasting snack. Nuts also help to reduce your risk of heart disease by lowering the bad LDL cholesterol. This is accomplished by the monounsaturated fats contained in nuts, which block the production and absorption of LDL cholesterol. Less bad cholesterol in the bloodstream equals less heart disease.

ALMONDS

Almonds are a tasty, crunchy, delicious snack, which are high in nutritional value. Almonds provide a good source of protein, fiber, vitamin E, and magnesium. Eating an ounce of healthful, monounsaturated almonds every day instead of foods which are higher in saturated fats, will actually lower your blood cholesterol. And, in addition to their great taste, they are filling and quickly suppress your appetite control mechanism so that you have no desire to snack on empty calories consisting of refined sugars and saturated fats. Almonds, along with most other nuts which are high in monounsaturated fats, are an excellent way to lose weight and stay healthy.

WALNUTS

Frequent consumption of nuts (four to five servings per week) has been shown to reduce the risk of coronary heart disease by as much as 50%. Nuts also have been shown to decrease both the total cholesterol by 5-10% and the LDL cholesterol by 15-20%. Several beneficial components of walnuts include L-arginine, which may be cardio-protective by dilating the arteries. Walnuts also contain fiber, folic acid, gamma-tocopherol, and other antioxidants, which also help to prevent arterio-sclerosis (hardening of the arteries).

A study published in the March 2002 issue of Journal of Nutrition indicated that of all edible plants, walnuts have one of the highest concentrations of antioxidants. In a more recent study reported in the April 6,

2004 issue of Circulation, from the Hospital Clinic of Barcelona, Spain, Dr. Emilio Ros said that, "This is the first time a whole food, not its isolated components, has shown this beneficial effect on vascular health." He further stated that, "Walnuts differ from all other nuts because of their high content of alpha-linolenic acid (ALA), a plant-based omega-3 fatty acid, which may provide additional heart-protective properties."

BEST NUTS

1. **Almonds**, ½ ounce – 12 nuts (80 calories, 7 grams of fat, and high in protein, magnesium, calcium, and vitamin E).
2. **Walnuts**, ½ ounce – 7 nuts (90 calories, 9 grams of fat, and high in omega-3 fatty acids and alpha-linoleic acid.
3. **Cashews**, ½ ounce – 10 nuts (80 calories, 6 grams of fat, and high in copper, magnesium, and iron).
4. **Hazelnuts**, ½ ounce – 10 nuts (85 calories, 8 grams of fat, and high in vitamin E, fiber, and iron).

GOOD NUTS

1. **Peanuts**, ½ ounce – 20 shelled (80 calories, 7 grams of fat, and high in protein, iron, and folate).
2. **Pecans**, ½ ounce – 10 nuts (93 calories, 10.2 grams of fat, and high in fiber, copper, and zinc).
3. **Pistachios**, ½ ounce – 23 nuts (78 calories, 6.3 grams of fat, and high in potassium, fiber, and protein).

WORST NUTS

1. **Macadamias**, ½ ounce – 5 nuts (102 calories, 105 grams of fat; much too high in total fat and calories).
2. **Chestnuts**, ½ ounce – 2 nuts (55 calories, 0.5 grams of fat, and some folate; even though they are low in calories and fat, they really have no heart health nutritious benefits).
3. **Brazil nuts**, ½ ounce – 4 nuts (90 calories, 9.5 grams of fat, and moderate levels of selenium and magnesium; there have been cases of Brazil nuts causing sickness due to contaminants and it is not a recommended healthy nut).

TIP # 35
BOOST ENERGY & CONTROL HUNGER

Protein is found in all of your body's cells. It is the essential nutrient that is responsible for the maintenance and repair of all of your organs, tissues, muscles, brain and bones. This individual built-in repair kit occurs at the cellular level in our bodies. Protein regulates everything from our blood circulation, our metabolism and our immune system. Individuals who lack sufficient protein in their bodies have weaker immune systems than people who consume adequate protein in their diets. Also, people who are constantly on yo-yo diets where they lose and gain weight back frequently usually become protein deficient and have weaker immune systems. This fact has been proven by researchers who have found that these yo-yo dieters have about a third lower the number of killer cell activity than normal individuals. The so-called killer blood cells are essential for the immune system to function properly.

All foods are sources of energy; however, protein provides a greater boost in energy levels since it is absorbed slowly and thus produces a constant source of energy. Protein has real energy-staying power for your active, healthy, lifestyle. Fats and carbohydrates produce quick bursts of energy but cannot be relied upon to provide the body with a continuous source of energy, since they are digested and metabolized more quickly than protein. Fats and carbohydrates also tend to be stored as fat in the body for later use. The protein that we're discussing is lean protein (lean meats, skinless poultry, seafood, egg whites, low-fat dairy products, legumes and beans, soy and tofu foods, skim and low-fat cheeses, and good-fat nuts). Lean proteins are also excellent sources of selenium, which is a mineral that protects the body against dangerous free radicals that can destroy normal cells in the body. These free radicals can damage many different types of cells including connective tissue, which causes joint and muscle inflammation.

High-saturated fat protein products like fatty meats, hard cheeses, whole fat milk dairy products, whole eggs, mayonnaise, luncheon and smoked meats including bacon, sausage, and hot dogs are definitely not good sources of energy production. The reason for this is, that even though these products have some protein content, its value is offset by the saturated fat content of these foods. The saturated fat content of these foods do more harm to the body (heart disease, strokes, hypertension, high cholesterol and some forms of cancer) than the protein portion of the food can repair. These are called harmful proteins and are not recommended for any healthful weight-loss program.

For appetite control, lean protein tops the charts for staying power. By adding a small portion of lean protein to your meal, you'll control hunger pangs for hours. Lean protein also has the advantage of being lower in calories than many foods, particularly saturated fat protein products, refined carbohydrates and saturated fat foods. Once you substitute saturated-fat protein products, you defeat the appetite-controlling factor of the protein. The fat content of saturated-fat protein foods prevents the brain's appetite-control center from shutting down. In other words, you'll get hungry soon after your meal of a saturated protein food.

Your body needs between 15-30% of its total daily calories from protein. To determine the number of grams of protein your body needs if you're fairly active, multiply your body weight in pounds by 0.5. For example, if you weigh 130 pounds, multiply that by 0.5 and you'll find that you need approximately 65 grams of protein daily for your body to function efficiently. If you're very active then you multiply your weight in pounds by 0.7, or if you're sedentary then multiply your body weight by 0.4. Eating too much protein, more than 35% of your total daily calories, however, can be dangerous, because it strains the kidneys. This is one of the reasons among many why low-carbohydrate, high saturated fat protein diets are dangerous to your health.

TIP # 36
ARE YOU A NIGHT EATER?

There is a condition called night eating syndrome or NES, which is actually a form of an eating disorder. These people actually wake up many times during the night and are unable to fall asleep unless they eat something, which is usually junk food, which then enables them to fall back to sleep. There is another documented night eating disorder, which is called sleep-related eating disorder or SRED. In this condition, people actually sleep walk to the kitchen for an eating binge. In both of these conditions, people eat mostly junk food, which can thwart attempts at staying on a balanced nutritious diet. These two types of night eating disorders also undermine good quality sleep. Both of these disorders actually require treatment by a physician.

However, there are milder variations of these disorders, which can keep many healthy people from continuing on a weight-loss program. Many people who are under stress may have some minor form of a night eating disorder, which causes them to eat lots of empty calories before bedtime or during the night. Others, however, often just develop a habit of night eating, which becomes very difficult to break. Most often the type of foods eaten are junk foods (cookies, doughnuts, cakes, etc.), which are high in calories, fat, and sugar. This immediate refined carbohydrate fix, which temporarily raises the blood sugar, causes these people to be able to fall asleep. However, oftentimes they awaken after the increase in insulin in their bloodstream occurs, which in turn causes a sudden drop in blood sugar, and causes them to wake up hungry again.

Aside from the two more serious eating disorders discussed above, the best remedy for most people who are night eaters and have either difficulty falling asleep or often wake up during the night and can't go back to sleep, is to have a **small lean high-protein snack**. For example, a slice of low-fat cheese, handful of nuts, glass of skim or soy milk, a cup of nonfat yogurt, or even a slice of turkey is all that is needed to satisfy the night eater's habit. These lean high-protein snacks are appetite satisfying, take longer to digest than carbohydrates, and help to break the junk food binging that night eaters so often engage in. Eating late in the evening, as long as it is a high-protein, low-calorie snack, will not cause you to gain weight just because you ate this snack at bedtime. Calories are calories, no matter when you consume them, and remember it's the total number of calories consumed in any 24-hour period that counts, not the time that you ate these calories. Binge eating, on the other hand, is the consumption of high-calorie, high-fat, high refined-sugar snacks that will certainly ruin any diet program and may, in fact, cause you to gain weight rather than lose weight.

If night eating can't be controlled by substituting lean high-protein snacks at night, then you certainly should consult with your physician to make sure that you do not have one of the more serious night eating disorders.

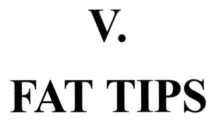

V.
FAT TIPS

TIP # 37
FATS – THE WORST & THE BEST!

Current guidelines for fat consumption are no more than 30% of total calories from fat. Most overweight or obese people consume twice that amount. Not only does this fat cause people to gain weight, but it also increases the risk for heart disease, stroke, diabetes, and high blood pressure.

Different foods contain many different types of fats, which can be described as being good, not so good, bad, or very bad fats. The following sections give a breakdown of the different types of fats.

Saturated fats are basically bad fats and are usually solid in nature, since the body uses them to produce other really bad fats called LDL cholesterol. This LDL cholesterol is what blocks your arteries and causes heart attacks, strokes, and diabetes. Saturated fats usually come from animal sources: meats, cheese, butter, milk, and other whole-milk dairy products. Some saturated fats are also found in tropical oils, such as coconut, cocoa butter, and palm kernel oils.

Polyunsaturated fats are usually liquid in nature. These fats, made from vegetables, include sunflower, cottonseed, safflower, and corn oils. In small amounts, they can help to reduce your cholesterol. However, taken in excess, these polyunsaturated oils can cause an inflammatory reaction in the body's tissues and prevent the immune system from working properly. These polyunsaturated fats may also be susceptible to oxidation, which then allows the cells to absorb bad fats (saturated fats and cholesterol). Here we have a case of a good fat turning bad.

Triglycerides are another type of fat that can be bad for you. If you eat excess amounts of refined sugar products (cakes, pies, candy, soda, baked goods, etc.), or eat a lot of fatty foods, or drink excessive amounts of alcohol, then the liver changes these excess calories into a form of fat known as triglycerides. Triglycerides have also recently been implicated in blocking the arteries to the heart and brain.

Trans fats

The really bad fats, and probably the worst fats that exist, are called trans fats. These fats are produced when the polyunsaturated fats in vegetable oils undergo a process called hydrogenation, where hydrogen atoms are added to the polyunsaturated fats. These very, very bad fats raise your blood levels of cholesterol and saturated fat, and lower your blood levels of your good HDL cholesterol. This type of bad fat is contained in foods such as baked goods, cookies, crackers, chips, margarine, and shortening. Avoid all products that say, "hydrogenated" or "partially hydrogenated" on the label. Unfortunately, the FDA will not be labeling the amount of trans fats contained in the foods you eat until 2006, so it is prudent to avoid all products that have hydrogenated or partially hydrogenated on the label.

Several new studies however, indicate that trans-fats can also increase the levels of a cellular component in the body, called *tumor necrosis factor.* This cellular component is considered a risk factor for diabetes, insulin resistance, coronary heart disease, heart failure and certain forms of cancer. It is thought that these conditions result from an inflammation that occurs in the body, caused by this tumor necrosis factor.

The following is a partial list of foods with high levels of trans-fats:
1. Margarine
2. Non-dairy creamers
3. Packaged cakes and cookies
4. Doughnuts and muffins
5. Frozen dinners
6. Cereal and energy bars
7. Crackers, chips and pretzels
8. Canned soups and sauces
9. Fast-foods (burgers, fries, & fried foods)
10. Mixes: pies, cakes and cookies

Food manufacturers started using trans fats in place of saturated fats in the mid-1980s. They thought that this type of fat would be healthier than saturated fat; however, it was discovered that these trans fats were as bad, if not worse, then the saturated fats that they initially used. These trans fats can raise the bad LDL cholesterol and lower the good HDL cholesterol. They also may increase the risk of heart attacks, strokes and diabetes. These trans fats were also added to foods to extend the shelf life of certain foods, much like preservatives are added to extend shelf life. These are very, very bad fats! Be very afraid!

Polyunsaturated fats, as we have seen previously, can be good in small to moderate amounts, but can turn really bad in large amounts. This is because of their content of ***omega-6 fatty acids.*** These omega-6 fatty acids are contained in vegetable oil, such as sunflower, safflower, corn, and cottonseed. These omega-6 fatty acids can help to lower blood cholesterol in small amounts. However, when you eat more polyunsaturated fats, you increase the absorption of omega-6 fatty acids in the bloodstream, which causes your cells to start to absorb more cholesterol and saturated fat. Here is another example of a good fat turned bad.

Monounsaturated fats are, by far, the best fats. These fats are liquid at room temperature. These really good fats can lower your total blood cholesterol, increase your good HDL cholesterol, and lower your bad LDL cholesterol. These good fats are found in olive oil, peanut oil, and canola oil. They should always be used, as substitutes for the potentially bad polyunsaturated fats, like corn, safflower, sunflower and cottonseed oils. The good monounsaturated fats are also found in most nuts and avocados.

TIP # 38
MAKE GOOD CHOICES!

1.   Limit beef to no more than once a week, since in addition to high levels of saturated fat, beef contains some nasty byproducts that can cause cancer and various forms of infectious disease. One infection in particular is caused by a small particle called a "prion," which has been thought to cause mad cow disease. Since prions are usually found in the brain and spinal cord, avoid sausages, hot dogs, and processed lunchmeats, which may also contain these deadly particles. It is advisable to also avoid what is called neck meat, and anything that is near the brain.

   a.   If you must eat meat, choose lean cuts of meat. "Prime grade" meat actually contains the highest amount of saturated fats. "Choice" meat is the next highest in fat content. Choose "Lean" meats or "Select" meats, which have a slightly lower fat content.
   b.   Avoid bacon, sausage, hot dogs, kielbasa, knockwurst, and high-fat lunchmeats, including liverwurst.
   c.   Always trim the fat from meats before cooking.
   d.   Avoid organ meats (brain, liver, kidney, thymus), which are very high in cholesterol and saturated fat.

2.   Chicken and turkey are good protein, low-fat substitutes for meat. Always remove the skin before cooking, since the fat content of the skin is absorbed during the cooking process. White meat has less fat than dark meat. If possible, choose free-range or organic chickens, which do not contain chemicals and hormones, which can be harmful to your body.

   a.   Low-fat turkey breast is a good meat substitute for sandwiches or salads.
   b.   Avoid breaded or fried chicken or chicken nuggets, which are particularly high in saturated fats.

    c. Avoid internal organs, such as liver, which again is very high in saturated fat.

3.   Fish is an excellent source of protein and contains the good *omega-3 fatty acids*. Fatty fish like tuna, salmon, sardines, herring, and haddock are particularly high in omega-3 fatty acids. Most fish are low in total saturated fats and cholesterol. Shellfish (shrimp, lobster, crab) are the exception, since they are high in cholesterol. However, shellfish are so low in total fat that the cholesterol content of shellfish is unlikely to raise your blood cholesterol.

    a. Always grill, broil, poach, or bake fish without breading. Add spices and lemon to enhance their flavors.

    b. Limit large fish intake, such as shark and swordfish and tile fish, since they may be higher in mercury content, particularly if you are pregnant or nursing.

4.   Dairy products

    a. Choose nonfat or 1% milk. 2% milk contains almost as much fat as does whole milk.

    b. Choose low-fat cheeses, like cottage cheese, goat cheese, skim milk mozzarella, and low-fat Swiss cheeses. Limit the high-fat processed cheeses, like American, cheddar, Brie, and Roquefort cheese.

    c. Egg whites are excellent sources of protein, without the cholesterol found in egg yolk; however, two to three whole eggs per week are not harmful and the yolk contains many nutrients beside cholesterol that are good for you. An egg white omelet or egg substitute omelet, with plenty of fresh veggies, is a healthful, low-fat, high-protein dish. Be sure to cook in a little olive oil, rather than butter or margarine.

    d. Butter is very high in saturated fat and margarine is just as bad for you, since it is high in polyunsaturated and trans fats. There are some newer butter substitutes on the market that are supposed to be heart-friendly. Use them sparingly.

e. Yogurt, sour cream, cream cheese are rich in protein and can be found in low or nonfat varieties. Always add fruit, when possible, to beef up the nutrient content.

f. Soy milk, tofu, and tempeh, all are rich in protein and contain plant nutrients. Many also contain isoflavones, which have estrogen-like qualities and can also have positive effects in menopausal symptoms and may help to lower blood fats.

5.   Fruits and vegetables are excellent low-fat, high-fiber foods. They contain many plant nutrients and can be freedom fighters against all sorts of degenerative diseases, including heart disease and cancer. They should always be included in any healthy diet plan.

TIP # 39
LOW FAT SNACKS

GRAINS
· Low-fat, low-sugar cereal bars (1).
· Low-fat, whole-wheat pretzels (2).
· Fat-free baked potato or corn chips without trans fats (handful).
· Rice cakes (1).
· Roasted peanuts in shell (handful).
· Low-fat or fat-free popcorn.
· Sunflower seeds (handful).
· Angel food cake (small slice) or a few gingersnap cookies.
· Handful of high-fiber, low-sugar cereal with or without skim milk.
· Peanut butter 1 Tbs. on 2-3 nonfat crackers.

FRUITS
· Raisins, grapes, strawberries, blueberries (1/2 cup).
· Wedges of oranges, grapefruit, or pineapple (1/2 cup).
· Dried fruits without added sugar (1/3 cup).
· Sliced bananas, pears, or apples (1).
· Pitted prunes (3-4).

VEGETABLES
· Celery or carrot sticks.
· Wedge of lettuce, broccoli, or cauliflower.
· Sliced cucumbers.
· Dip above in nonfat dip or salsa.

DAIRY (1/2 cup of each)
· Nonfat yogurt with or without fruit topping.
· Skim milk (1 glass).

·   Fat-free cottage cheese or sour cream with or without fruit topping.
·   Nonfat, low-sugar ice cream.

SWEET TOOTH SNACKS
·   Low-fat peppermint patties (1 small).
·   Frozen sherbert, yogurt, or juice bar (1/2 bar).
·   Fat-free ice cream sandwich (1/2).
·   Jellybeans (6).
·   Sugar-free hard candies made for diabetics (4).

DRINKS
·   Diet soda, iced tea or coffee (decaffeinated).
·   Bottled water (six 8-oz. bottles daily).
·   Skim milk (1-2 glasses per day).
·   Vegetable juice without added sugar (one 8-oz. glass).
·   Nonfat latte or cappuccino with skim milk and no whipped cream. Add small amount of mocha, if desired.
·   Protein shake with 1 cup of skim milk or yogurt plus fruit of choice. For protein boost, add 1 Tbs. of wheat germ or whey protein.

TOPPINGS
·   Fat-free whipped cream for fruits (small amount).
·   Fat-free salad dressings and salsa for salads and vegetable snacks.
·   Fat-free fudge (1 Tbs.).

TIP # 40
FAT MAKES YOU FAT!

The American diet has a higher fat content than almost any other country in the world. This increased fat intake in our diet is responsible for the development of *obesity*, as well as many other disorders. Fat is the most concentrated source of calories, since a gram of dietary fat supplies your body with *nine calories*. This is compared to only four calories per gram of protein or carbohydrate. Since fat has this concentrated source of calories, it is the *most fattening* type of food that we consume. When you reduce fat calories, you reduce your total calorie content significantly which results in more weight lost.

In a study just released by the National Heart, Lung and Blood Institute in Bethesda, Maryland, obesity has now been listed as a major independent risk factor for heart disease. What's so new about that? Everyone knows that being overweight contributes to heart disease. That's just it; up until now obesity was just a contributing factor in heart disease because of its relationship with high blood pressure and high cholesterol. Now, it has gained it own independent rating as causing heart disease all by itself. This study followed 5,000 women and men for 26 years. The risk of developing heart disease was found to be more pronounced in people who gained most of their excess weight after the age of 25. One important point made in this extensive study was that *losing a moderate amount of weight lessened the risk of developing heart disease.*

Since fat has the most concentrated source of calories (9 calories per gram), it is the most fattening type of food that you can consume. Therefore, cutting down on the total fat intake in your diet is one of the best ways to cut down on the total amount of calories that you consume, in order to lose weight. Controlling your weight by reducing the amount of saturated fat in your diet has a two-fold benefit. First of all, it will help to control and maintain your weight. Secondly, it will have the beneficial effect of helping to prevent heart attacks and strokes, since these illnesses have been associated with high levels of blood cholesterol, which result from the consumption of saturated fats.

Weight gain actually occurs from taking in more calories in the form of dietary fats than were burned off as a fuel for energy. On a low-fat diet, calories are removed from storage in fat cells and are added to the fuel mixture of protein and carbohydrate for the production of energy. This results in steady, permanent weight loss, unlike the temporary water weight loss of low-carbohydrate diets. The equation is simple: Less fat taken in results in more storage fat being burned as fuel. More fat taken in results in more fat being stored and less fat being burned, which causes fatty deposits in the abdomen, buttocks, thighs and hips. In other words, *it's the fat in your diet that makes you fat!*

Since one pound of body fat contains 3,500 calories; therefore, it stands to reason, that the only way to lose one pound of body weight is to burn 3500 calories. This can only be accomplished by cutting back on the total amount of fat calories in your diet and also by increasing your physical activity. Nothing else works! One of my favorite sayings to my patients when they ask me how to lose weight is, "The only way you can really lose weight is to eat less fat and walk more, or if you would like, you can walk more and eat less fat!"

TIP # 41
WHAT ARE LIPIDS ANYWAY?

The term lipids is used to include all fats and fat-like substances that circulate in our bloodstreams. These lipids however, will not dissolve in water and are therefore called fat-soluble substances. So how do these fats get absorbed into the bloodstream, since the blood is a water-soluble solution? These lipids have to hook up with certain proteins in our blood so that they can dissolve in water (in this case the blood) and now become known as lipoproteins (fat & protein combinations). The two main types of lipids in the blood that are combined with proteins are cholesterol and triglycerides. These lipoprotein combinations are classified on the basis of their density in the blood stream.

1.   CHOLESTEROL:

Cholesterol is an essential element of all animal cell membranes and forms the structure of the body's hormones and bile acids. However, when cholesterol levels get too high in our blood streams they can become very dangerous. There are three important types of cholesterol that you have to consider for good health.

a.   Total Cholesterol is the total amount of cholesterol circulating in your blood. This number is derived by the total amount of cholesterol and fat that you eat, combined with the amount of cholesterol manufactured by your liver.

b.   LDL Cholesterol (low-density lipoprotein) is referred to as the bad cholesterol. This type of cholesterol is the type most likely to clog up your arteries and cause heart attacks and strokes. This LDL cholesterol comes primarily from eating excess saturated fats and cholesterol-laden foods. Following a low-fat, high-fiber diet combined with regular exercise can usually lower this LDL cholesterol. In many people however, LDL cholesterol can be genetic and has little or nothing to do with your diet. In these particular cases, someone slipped you a bad cholesterol gene and often times the LDL can only be lowered by cholesterol-lowering medications prescribed by your physician.

  c. HDL Cholesterol (high-density lipoprotein) is called the good cholesterol. The HDL cholesterol acts opposite the bad cholesterol, by helping to prevent the formation of cholesterol deposits that form in your arteries. It accomplishes this by collecting the excess amounts of bad cholesterol in the blood before it has a chance to clog up your arteries. It then transports this bad cholesterol to the liver, where it is eliminated from the body. There have been recent medical reports that show that the HDL cholesterol can actually shovel the bad cholesterol out of the cholesterol deposits (plaques) that have already formed in the arteries. Pretty cool!

  Well, how do we get some of this good cholesterol? As always however, there's got to be a catch. First and foremost, heredity plays an important role in the body's production of this good cholesterol. Some people have more HDL than others simply because of good genes. Secondly, cutting saturated fats and cholesterol from our diets has little to do with raising HDL cholesterol. However, adding the heart-healthy monounsaturated fats such as olive oil and nuts, and the omega-3 fatty acids found in fish like salmon and tuna have been shown to raise the HDL cholesterol. A regular moderate intensity exercise, such as walking, can also help to raise the good cholesterol, whereas the lack of exercise and smoking will considerably lower the good cholesterol. Individuals who cannot raise their good (HDL) cholesterol and can't lower their bad (LDL) cholesterol by diet and exercise, often have to take the cholesterol-lowering medications under a doctor's supervision.

2. TRIGLYCERIDES:

  Triglycerides are the major lipids transported in the blood. The triglycerides are the least dense of the fat and protein combinations and are called very low-density lipoproteins (VLDL). Triglycerides are important in transferring energy from the food that we eat into your body's cells and consequently they help to regulate your cells' metabolism.

Excess amounts of triglycerides in the blood often lead to diabetes, glucose intolerance, obesity, gout and coronary artery disease. Some cases of high blood triglycerides are genetic while many others are the result of eating too many refined carbohydrates, sugars, saturated fats and alcohol. The most important way to control high triglycerides in the blood is to restrict the amount of refined carbohydrates, sugars and saturated fats that you eat and to limit the amount of alcoholic beverages that you consume. Many people with this condition go on to develop diabetes and heart disease when this condition is left untreated. A high-fiber diet consisting of whole grain cereals and breads, legumes and beans, and fruits and vegetables has been shown to lower high serum triglycerides. A regular aerobic exercise program like walking has also been shown to lower blood triglycerides. However, like with blood cholesterol, there are some cases that cannot be lowered with diet and exercise and have to be treated with medication by your physician.

Several recent studies have shown that it may actually be your triglycerides and not your will-power that are to blame for overeating. It seems that people with high blood triglycerides were shown to have difficulty in curbing their appetites. This appears to be due to the fact that high blood levels of triglycerides block the formation of an appetite-controlling hormone called *leptin*. This condition sets up a vicious cycle, since the more refined sugars and saturated fats that you eat, the higher your blood levels of triglycerides become. And these high triglycerides shut down the production of the appetite controlling hormone leptin and subsequently you don't feel full when in actuality you are really full. So what do you do next? Eat more refined sugars and saturated fats. The only way to break this overeating cycle is to severely restrict your refined sugars and saturated fats in the first place. Then your triglycerides do not become abnormally elevated and your appetite controlling hormone leptin is not blocked. So when you eat and become full you will actually feel full and stop eating at the appropriate time.

TIP # 42
CHOLESTEROL CONTENT OF FOODS

MEAT, FISH, AND POULTRY HIGH IN CHOLESTEROL

Fatty cuts of beef, pork, ham, veal, and mutton	Luncheon meats and canned meats; sausage
Duck, goose	Sardines, herring
Organ meats, (kidney, liver, heart, sweetbread, and brain)	Shellfish (shrimp, lobster, crab, clams, oysters, scallops)

Although high in cholesterol, shellfish are low in saturated fat and should not be restricted on a weight-loss program.

MEAT, FISH, AND POULTRY LOW IN CHOLESTEROL

Chicken and turkey without skin	Tuna and salmon packed in water or with oil drained
Fresh fish (flounder, cod, bass, sole, perch, haddock, halibut, salmon, trout, tuna, carp, pike)	Lean ground meat and very lean cuts of beef, pork, ham, and veal

DAIRY PRODUCTS HIGH IN CHOLESTEROL

Whole milk	Creams (sour, whipped, half & half, ice cream, and cheeses made from whole milk or cream)
Evaporated milk	Eggs
Cheeses	Butter

DAIRY PRODUCTS LOW IN CHOLESTEROL

Nonfat or skimmed milk	Low-fat yogurt
Low-fat buttermilk	Cocoa
Canned evaporated nonfat milk	Cheeses made from skimmed milk
Margarines high in polyunsaturates	Egg whites
Egg substitutes (Fleischmann's Egg Beaters®)	Low-fat cheeses
Low-fat cottage cheese	Low-fat sour cream

BREAD AND CEREAL HIGH IN CHOLESTEROL

Commercial muffins	Rolls and buns
Biscuits & butter rolls	Coffee cakes
Donuts	Crackers & croissants
Mixes containing whole milk, butter, and eggs	White bread, Italian and French bread
Corn bread & garlic bread	Granola cereals

BREAD AND CEREAL LOW IN CHOLESTEROL

Whole-wheat, pumpernickel, rye, and cracked wheat breads	Cereals, hot and cold (whole-grain and bran type, served with low-fat milk)
Homemade cookies, muffins, and biscuits, if made with olive or canola oil and egg whites	English muffins (oats, bran or whole wheat)
Bread sticks & rice cakes	Bran muffins (non-fat)
Matzo, soda crackers	Whole wheat pita

DESSERTS AND SNACKS HIGH IN CHOLESTEROL

Commercial pies	Whipped cream
Pastries	Ice cream

Cookies	Fried foods
Cake	Snack foods
Puddings	Coconut
Cocoa butter	Potato and corn chips

DESSERTS AND SNACKS LOW IN CHOLESTEROL

Home-baked pastries and pies (made with nonfat milk, liquid olive or canola oil, and egg whites)	Cookies, cakes, and puddings made with monounsaturated oil and nonfat milk
Commercial gelatins	Honey, marmalade
Sherbert, non-fat ice cream or frozen yogurt	Non-fat hard or soft pretzels (ex. Superpretzel®)
Jelly, jam	Angel food cake
Nuts, fruits and vegetables	Pure peanut butter (made with egg white only)

OTHER FOODS LOW IN CHOLESTEROL

Most fish (except shellfish); however, shellfish are low in total saturated fat and are fine for a weight-loss program	Chick peas, soybeans, lentils, and baked beans (Since dried beans and peas are high in protein and low in cholesterol, they can be substituted for meat)
Pastas, noodles, and rice – whole-grain types	Beverages include tea, coffee, carbonated drinks
Raw or cooked vegetables, without sauces or butter or margarine	Fruits and vegetables – fresh, frozen, or canned, with no sugar or syrup added

TIP # 43
BURN FAT CALORIES

1. When shopping, go to the market after you've eaten, so you won't buy impulse high-fat snack foods. Buy only items on a prepared list that you make before marketing. Don't deviate from this list with snack foods, which you might have a tendency to buy if you had not eaten prior to marketing.

2. When shopping for packaged or canned goods, make sure the item of food you are purchasing has no more than 1.5-2.0 grams of total fat. If it is higher, look for another brand. Always look for nonfat or low-fat products; however, remember to look at the label, and don't depend on a label that says low-fat food. Many so-called low-fat items are fairly high in total fat content; for example, 2% milk has 5 grams of fat, or 98% fat-free yogurt can have 3.5-4.0 grams of total fat. Always choose foods that are less than 2.0 grams of total fat. These foods may have 0 grams of cholesterol; however, they may contain many grams of total fat.

3. Don't use foods as a stress reliever. Most people have a tendency to seek out high-fat, high-sugar foods when under stress. Substitute music, exercise, meditation, or a warm bath for food cravings.

4. Make your meals attractive with colorful foods, garnishes and greens, carrots, tomatoes, broccoli, spinach, peppers, yams, celery, parsley, etc., in order to make them more appealing, and vary your meal plans daily to avoid boredom. Remember that the more colorful the foods are, the more phytonutrients they contain.

5. Foods should be kept out of sight between meals, in your refrigerator or pantry.

6. People who skip breakfast usually wind up with a high-fat, high-sugar snack (example, doughnut and coffee mid-morning). A high-fiber, low-fat cereal with fruit and skim milk will hold you comfortably until lunchtime.

7. Fresh vegetables and fruits are better choices than canned fruits and vegetables, which can be loaded with salt or sugar.

8.   Soups and stews can be loaded with hidden fats. Refrigerate them overnight after preparing, and skim off the layer of fat that is lying on the surface of the stew or soup. You'll be removing more than 3/4 of the fat contained in these products. Choose soups loaded with vegetables and beans, and avoid any soups that are cream-based.

9.   Drink at least six 8-ounce glasses of water daily. Avoid drinking a lot of artificially sweetened drinks, as they can increase your appetite due to the hypoglycemic effect (they lower your blood sugar).

10.   Cream, whole milk, or powdered creamers should be avoided in coffee or tea. Substitute skim milk. Non-fat dairy creamers may contain trans-fats. Check for the words "hydrogenated or partially hydrogenated" on ingredient labels.

11.   Low-fat, nonfat, or part-skim milk cheeses should be substituted for all other cheese. Make sure, however, that you check the total fat content per serving size. Low fat goat cheese, feta, mozerella and ricotta cheese are good choices.

12.   Baked potato with the skin is an excellent food for meals or snacks (high fiber, low fat), compared to French fries, which are saturated with up to 15 grams of fat per serving. However, if you have a craving for French fries, you can prepare low-fat French fries by slicing potatoes, spraying with nonfat vegetable spray, and baking for 20-30 minutes in an oven at approximately 350°, or microwaving for 3-5 minutes. Keep your portion size small.

13.   Use a rack to roast meat, poultry, or fish. The fat drips off during cooking. Baste with broth or vegetable juice to preserve moisture. Never use butter, margarine, shortening, or gravy mixes. Defatted chicken broth is a good alternative.

14.   Trim all visible skin and fat from poultry and meat before cooking.

15.   Fresh or canned beans of any variety are excellent sources of fiber and vitamins. Their low fat content makes them excellent companions to any meal. Make sure they are not prepared with meat (example: baked beans with bacon). Avoid

high-fat, refried beans; however, several companies now have nonfat refried beans available.

16. Fruit and vegetable skins are excellent sources of fiber, as well as the seeds (berries, tomatoes, cucumbers, and pumpkins).

17. Avoid sugar in sodas, teas, and fruit drinks. Use fresh orange juice, grapefruit juice, tomato juice (low sodium), and non-caffeinated teas, coffee, and sodas for snack drinks. Make plain old water (tap or bottled) your drink of choice. Remember to drink at least six 8-ounce glasses of water daily.

18. Skim milk, which has no fat, has all of the calcium, vitamins, and minerals that are present in 1%, 2%, or whole milk, and it tastes just as good.

19. Nonfat yogurt is an excellent source of calcium, and its lacto-bacillus and other cultures are friendly bacteria for your colon.

20. Breads that are high in fiber, low in fat, are the following: whole grain, bran enriched, cracked wheat, whole-wheat pita, rye, pumpernickel, and those labeled high fiber breads. High-fat, low-fiber breads are French, Italian, white, garlic bread and rolls. Stay away from them. Remember to check the ingredients label. If the first ingredient doesn't say "whole-grain," then it is not a whole-grain, high-fiber bread.

TIP # 44
LOW FAT DIET TIPS

1. A tasty nonfat dessert is angel food cake with fresh fruit and nonfat whipped cream. (A slice of cheese or chocolate cake has up to 14 grams of fat). The angel food cake, as described above, has less than 1.5 grams of fat.

2. Sherbert, sorbet, frozen fruit bars, and nonfat frozen yogurts are excellent substitutes for your ice cream sweet tooth.

3. Salad dressing and mayonnaise are no-no's in a low fat diet plan. Substitute nonfat dressings or nonfat mayonnaise. If not available, use either no dressing or just dip your fork gently into the dressing on the side every 2-3 bites of salad, and you'll get the taste without the added fat calories.

4. Nonfat popcorn is an excellent low-fat, high-fiber snack. Don't add butter or salt. Use hot air popper or microwave nonfat varieties.

5. When eating out, choose low-fat foods without sauces, like broiled fish or chicken, with a large tossed salad. Avoid excess alcohol, since it can increase your appetite and add extra calories. Incidentally, one gram of alcohol contains 7 calories, higher than a gram of carbohydrate or protein. If you definitely like a drink with dinner, a wine spritzer is a good substitute, which is relatively low in total calorie value. However, 4 ounces of red wine or a light beer is permitted three times per week.

6. At parties, weddings, etc., concentrate on the fresh vegetables, without the dips, and fresh fruits. Avoid those fat-laden little appetizers with toothpicks in them. They're red flags warning you to stay away!

7. When traveling by air, order ahead for a low-fat meal when making reservations. They're available! Otherwise, if it is a short flight, have a low-fat snack prior to boarding.

8. Nonstick pans use less fat than cast iron, copper, or aluminum pans. Use nonstick vegetable sprays as the first choice; otherwise, a small amount of olive oil (1 tsp.) or canola oil can be used for cooking.

9. Grilled or broiled foods, which include vegetables, fish, poultry, and lean meats, are tasty low-fat dishes. The fat drips away as the foods are cooked.

10. Steamed vegetables, with or without herbs, can be cooked in a basket over boiling water. Steaming retains the flavor, color, and nutrients of the vegetable.

11. Poaching fish in water at a simmer (just below the boiling point of water) preserves the taste and texture of the fish. Any condiments can be added to the liquid to enhance the flavor, such as garlic or herbs.

12. Stir-frying in a pan or wok is a fast way to make tasty vegetables, chicken, meats, or fish. Add very small amounts of olive or peanut oil and seasonings, followed by either defatted chicken broth or low-sodium soy sauce.

13. Sautéing: Use nonstick, nonfat vegetable sprays or a small amount of wine or defatted broth. Vegetables, fish, poultry, or meats are mixed together in a pan. Then add herbs, such as thyme, basil, sage, or dill, for added taste.

14. Microwaving food uses the food's own moisture to cook. It's quick and easy, and you don't have to add any fat when microwaving. Almost all foods are microwaveable.

15. Peeling a potato (white or sweet potato) before cooking or eating removes more than 25% of its nutrients and 35-40% of its fiber.

16. If you put salt on poultry, fish, or meat before cooking, the food loses a good portion of its vitamin and mineral content during the cooking process. This is because the added salt causes the food to be drained of its nutrients during the cooking process, which then end up in the cooking broth.

17. Don't be afraid to send back your meal in a restaurant if they didn't follow your instructions for your order. For example,

if you asked for steamed vegetables, baked potato, and broiled fish without butter, that's the way it should arrive on your plate.

18. Pasta: Spaghetti or linguini is lower in fat than wider pastas that are often made with eggs. Try to order (restaurant) or buy whole-grain pasta or spinach noodles for their high fiber content. Stick to tomato or marinara sauces (some, however, have too much oil, and you can have the waiter drain the oil from the pasta and bring back your dish), or seafood-based sauces, without cream, are also good substitutes.

19. Pizza can be ordered without cheese (tomato pie) and then add on a variety of fresh vegetables. If you want cheese, sprinkle on a little Parmesan cheese. **Tip:** Always blot a cheese pizza with a couple of napkins before eating, to remove the extra oil and fat.

20. Chinese restaurants: Stir-fry foods are better than deep-fried. Choose dishes with grains and vegetables. Order brown rice instead of white rice for the extra fiber content (not fried rice, which also comes out brown in color, but is low in fiber). Ask to have your food prepared without soy sauce or MSG. Choose vegetable wonton soup or any vegetable-based soup, rather than meat-based soups.

21. Mexican foods are great, if you can stay away from the deep-fried tortilla chips and order oven-baked chips with salsa instead. Skip the sour cream and go light on the guacamole (avocado), both of which are high in fat. Soft corn tortillas (tostados or enchiladas) with chicken, tomato sauce, and onions are good low-fat choices. Burritos or fajitas without sour cream or guacamole are excellent choices, with lettuce, tomato, and onion, and can be considered low-fat dishes. Avoid regular refried beans, deep-fried chimichangas, beef taco salad, and deep-fried tortilla chips.

22. Choose whole-wheat or oat bran English muffins, whole-wheat bread, whole-wheat or oat bran bagels or raisin bread instead of sweet rolls, doughnuts, cakes, and white bread.

23. Fat-free snack: Dried or fresh fruits, raisins, peaches, apples, plums, apricots, and bananas.

24. Non-fat hard pretzels and non-fat soft pretzels (Superpretzel®), rice cakes (flavored), or hot-air popped corn are excellent low-fat snacks.
25. Spread for breads: Jelly, honey, fruit preserves and all-fruit jams instead of margarine or butter.
26. Baked potatoes with skin or corn chips (nonfat) in place of French fries or potato chips.

TIP # 45
BEWARE THE HIDDEN FATS!

Fat accounted for approximately 30% of our calories in the early 1900s, whereas today, the fat content of our diet has more than 40% of our calories coming from fat. In order to meet the basic nutritional requirements, we need only eat 1 Tbs. of *polyunsaturated oil* each day, which supplies the essential fatty acid called *linoleic acid*. This essential fatty acid helps you absorb fat-soluble vitamins. Americans, however, eat six to eight times this amount of fat, and fat can be considered to be the major source of nutritionally empty calories for most Americans.

Americans have become more conscious of fat consumption in the past ten years; however, only about one-third of the fat we eat is *visible* fat, such as hard fat on meat, fats and oils used in cooking, and oil-based salad dressings. Most of the fat in our diet, unfortunately, is hidden fat and not as readily noticeable as the marbled fat on meat. *Hidden fat*, unfortunately, is a major part of hard cheeses, cream cheese, deep-fried foods, creamed soups, ice cream, chocolate, nuts, and seeds. Hidden fat is also a major ingredient of processed, prepared foods, such as baked goods (pies, cakes, and cookies), processed meats (bologna, hot dogs, etc.), coffee creamers, whipped toppings, snack foods, and instant meals. Many health food products that are purchased as substitutes for saturated fats have in themselves high fat content. Nuts and seeds, sesame paste, granola, quiches, and avocados may contain more than half the calories as fat calories. However, nuts and avocados contain the heart-healthy monounsaturated fats.

When shopping in the market, it is often difficult to tell how much fat is contained in processed foods. Always check the label for the ingredients and remember that the ***ingredients are listed in order of their weight***. Therefore, if fat or oil is listed as one of the first two ingredients, then the product is likely to be high in fat, especially if it precedes the flour content; for example, in baked goods. The **Nutritional Facts label** will tell you how much total fat and saturated fat is in each serving, and what the serving size is.

Trans fats (bad fats) aren't listed, since there is no current requirement to label trans-fatty acids in food products. Trans fat is produced when unsaturated fat is hydrogenated, turning it into a solid. Next, check the *Ingredients* label. If *hydrogenated or partially hydrogenated fat* is listed, then a pretty good estimate is to consider that in most hydrogenated food products, the trans fat content probably equals the amount of saturated fat on the label. So, if 2 grams of saturated fat is listed on the label, you can double that amount, making it 4 grams per serving.

FATS

Whipped margarine and butter contain less fat per serving than regular margarine or butter because air or water replaces some of the fat in these products. A tablespoon of mayonnaise or oil may have as many fat calories as a teaspoon of hard fat; however, the softer, more liquid fats are less saturated. It is far better to choose the newer soft spreads that are labeled oil-free, which contain no trans fats.

DAIRY PRODUCTS

Low-fat, 1% milk or skim milk is preferable to any other milk product. Low-fat yogurt, cottage cheese, and ricotta cheese are preferable to other dairy products. Parmesan, feta and mozzarella cheese made from skim milk have less fat than hard cheeses. Sour cream and sweet cream both are high in fat content and should be avoided. Use skim milk if you are preparing puddings or custards from a packaged mix. Non-fat ice cream and frozen yogurt have less fat than ice cream and milkshakes. Soft ice cream, such as frozen custard, may contain as much fat as the hard varieties. Buttermilk contains little or no butterfat and can be used in baked goods to add taste and richness.

SALADS

Salads are fine for a low-fat diet, provided they are made without dressings. Use herbs and spices instead. Occasionally adding lemon juice with the spices will be satisfactory. There are also low calorie salad dressings, which can be used; however, they, too, have a considerable fat content. The newer nonfat salad dressings are preferable, as well as the monounsaturated olive oil.

SOUPS

Clear consommé broth and clear soup made with noodles, beans, rice, or vegetables, are preferable to creamed soups or heavy stock soups.

MEATS

Heavily marbled prime cuts of meats and processed meats are the highest in fat content. Sirloin tip, London broil, and flank steak are leaner than heavily marbled beef. Veal and leg of lamb are also lean. Always buy lean hamburger. Never fry meats; always broil or grill. Avoid gravies and cream sauces. Make gravy at home, after skimming off the fat. Limit meat intake to once or twice a week and always keep portion sizes small.

FISH

Tuna and salmon, surprisingly, are among the fattier fishes. However, they contain the heart-protective omega-3 fatty acids that are good for you. Sardines in oil and many forms of smoked fish are also high in fat content. Fresh fish, in particular flounder, cod, halibut, perch, haddock, and sole, have considerably less fat. Tuna packed in water has approximately one-third the fat content of tuna packed in oil. Shellfish, surprisingly, although having a high cholesterol content, are low in saturated fats, and will not raise your blood cholesterol when used in moderation.

POULTRY

Poultry should also be broiled or grilled, rather than fried. Discard the skin of poultry, preferably before cooking, so as to avoid the saturated fats being absorbed into the carcass of the poultry. Do not use creamed sauces or gravies. Always trim off skin before eating any poultry product.

VEGETABLES

Vegetables, fortunately, are a low source of dietary fat. In many cases, they can be substituted for protein because of the protein content of many vegetable products. Dried beans, legumes, peas, kidney beans, split peas, lentils, and bean curd are particularly high in fiber content and low in fat, and of moderate protein value. Nuts, soy and tofu foods are also excellent sources of protein. All other vegetables and fruits are without saturated fat content and are excellent sources of complex carbohydrates for the body.

BAKED GOODS

Commercially prepared baked goods contain considerable saturated fat. The one exception to this is angel food cake. Sweetened fig bars, vanilla wafers, and gingersnaps have less fat than cookies and cakes made with chocolate or cream fillings. Remember to check labels for "partially hydrogenated oils." These are the so-called *trans fats*, and they can raise your blood cholesterol. If hydrogenated or partially hydrogenated oils appear in the ingredients, you can double the amount of saturated fat listed on the label. Biscuits, muffins, croissants, and butter rolls are high in fat content. English muffins, French or Italian breads are lower in fat content; however, whole-wheat, whole-grain breads are best. Bread sticks, matzos, and rice cakes are low-fat substitutes for most potato chips and crackers, which are high in fat content.

TIP # 46
MELT BELLY FAT!

People whose diets are high in saturated fats are prone to storing fat in the abdomen, which surround vital organs, such as the liver, pancreas and intestinal tract. This type of fat is referred to as visceral fat and puts these individuals at risk for developing diabetes, fatty liver and heart disease. This abdominal or visceral fat is the direct result of eating saturated fats such as fatty meats, deli meats, cheeses, butter, whole milk products, and pre-packaged foods made with hydrogenated or partially hydrogenated oils and containing the bad trans-fats. Unfortunately, in some cases, genetics plays a role in developing excess abdominal fat. In these cases you should make an extra effort to limit saturated fat products to no more than 10 % of your total daily calorie intake. In those individuals who have the genetic trait for developing excessive abdominal fat and also have high levels of blood fats no matter how hard they try to diet, a physician should be consulted for the possibility of taking a cholesterol lowering medication.

Often the last place that you've gained weight is the first place that the weight will come off when you cut the saturated fat out of your diet. So if you start to gain abdominal fat you may notice that you'll lose inches around your middle, when you start your low fat diet. When you reduce your fat and calorie intake, you will lose weight all over your body including that unsightly belly fat.

Walk Off Belly Fat

Even though there is no magic diet for getting rid of abdominal fat, there is an easy solution to the problem. An aerobic exercise such as walking is the secret formula that can strengthen your abdominal muscles and help you to lose abdominal fat. As you swing your upper arms while walking, the upper chest wall muscles that are tied into your abdominal muscles will tighten and help to give you a flat, firm tummy without any additional exercises such as sit-ups.

First of all, when you walk briskly with an even stride, you are contracting and relaxing muscles in your chest, back, and abdomen. With each forward motion of your legs, these muscles contract to keep your body erect. Your abdominal muscles tighten automatically, exactly as they would if you were doing strenuous sit-ups, with one exception – you're not straining your back! As you walk, your upper body chest wall muscles aid in tightening the lower abdominal muscles. This combination of upper body and lower abdominal muscle contractions is what produces *a firm, flat tummy.*

Walking regularly tightens abdominal muscles and helps to burn away belly fat and as an added bonus it will also help to trim down your hips, thighs and buttocks. Since walking is a moderate aerobic exercise, it burns fat rather than carbohydrates. When this walking fat-burning exercise is combined with light hand-held weights (see Tips #96 & 97), you can speed up the abdominal flattening process as you burn fat and build muscle. Inactivity is what leads to the accumulation of fatty deposits in the abdomen and the loss of connective tissue elasticity.

Melt Belly Fat Faster

Refined carbohydrates that we eat are gradually absorbed into the blood stream, which causes a sudden spike in insulin production. This excess amount of insulin in our blood causes these digestive refined carbohydrates to head straight into our fat cells, particularly our belly's fat cells. This is due to the fact that the fat cells in the belly are located close to the digestive tract and also because the abdomen contains the most concentrated number of fat cells in the body. Once the excess insulin has done its work of dropping the blood sugar and packing fat into your fat cells, the low blood sugar that results, causes another round of carbohydrate cravings. It's like a lose-lose combination.

As we age, we crave more carbohydrates, and the more carbs we eat, the more calories become stored as fat in our abdomens. Due to certain hormonal changes which regulate our digestive system, we become less able to burn carbs as fuel, thus making carbs more likely to become stored as fat. This becomes a vicious cycle, because the more carbs we store as belly fat actually cause an increase in our craving for more carbohydrates. Stored abdominal fat suppresses the formation of a fat-burning hormone called *leptin*, which helps to keep blood sugar steady. Consequently, the more abdominal fat that you store, the easier it becomes to gain more weight, because less leptin is being produced and subsequently less fat is being burned.

If you can lose abdominal fat, then you will diminish carbohydrate cravings, and subsequently lose the unwanted belly fat. By eating *high fiber foods*, you can actually block the absorption of refined carbohydrates and starches. This is accomplished since the high fiber foods prevent the absorption of these refined carbohydrates by forming a web or network of fibers, which encircle these starches. This fiber web actually carries the starches out of the digestive tract almost completely intact and undigested. By blocking most of the absorption of these refined starches, less sugar and insulin are present in the blood stream, which results in less craving for carbohydrates. Less craving for carbohydrates results in more belly fat being burned and subsequently more weight being lost, particularly around the abdomen.

Some high fiber foods, particularly beans (white, kidney, fava, chick peas), contain an *enzyme-blocking compound*, which blocks pancreatic enzymes (amylase and lipase) from breaking down refined starches. By inhibiting these pancreatic enzymes from absorbing refined carbohydrates, your digestive tract bypasses the absorption of these starches and transports them out of the digestive tract as though they were never totally digested. This results in a much slower rise in blood sugar, which in turn doesn't cause a spike in insulin production and consequently reduces your craving for carbohydrates. This results in less fat stored in your belly.

Tip: According to a new study from Tufts University in Boston, people who eat too much white bread have larger waistlines than those individuals who eat whole grains. White bread appears to go straight to your abdomen and is stored as belly fat. People who ate the most white bread were also the fattest and had a higher risk of heart disease, compared to those who didn't carry the extra weight around the belly.

VI.
GREAT
WEIGHT-LOSS
TIPS

TIP # 47
THE ULTIMATE DIET FOOD

Two-thirds of our body is made up of water. Water is essential for our very existence, since it transports nutrients and oxygen though the blood stream to all of your body's cells and removes toxins and waste products from our body's tissues. Water regulates our body's temperature and metabolism, and aids in the digestion of all of the food we ingest. Water also provides the lubrication that makes our muscles and joints move efficiently and effortlessly.

Drinking water fuels the body's energy level, since the body's metabolic process requires a constant supply of water to function properly and efficiently. Your body actually loses water all of the time, just by the daily activity of living, whether you're active or sedentary. So you need to replenish your body with water constantly in order to replenish those losses.

Water is the ultimate diet food since it contains no calories and satisfies your hunger quickly. Many people who think they're hungry are in fact actually dehydrated. When your stomach is empty it is often the result of a lack of both food and water. Starting every meal with a glass of water is the best way to satisfy your appetite before you eat and it will keep you from eating excess calories at each meal. Water is also the best way to keep your appetite in check between meals.

Most studies show that for good health you should drink between 60-75 ounces of water daily. A good rule of thumb is to drink ½ your weight in ounces daily. For example, if you weigh 140 pounds, you should drink 70 ounces of water daily. This daily amount of water is the amount that is needed just for normal daily hydration. For exercise on the other hand, the amount of additional water needed for proper hydration increases with the level of intensity of the activity. To prevent dehydration, you should drink 1-½ cups of water 30 minutes before your exercise. Drink an additional 1-cup of water for each 15 minutes that you exercise moderately and 2 cups of water for each 15 minutes of severe exercise where you perspire excessively.

The best sources of water are of course portable bottled water. Sodas, juices, coffee and other beverages are also good sources of water. Stay away from caffeine whenever possible since it can speed up your metabolism and burn more water in your body. Alcohol is definitely not the liquid of choice for hydration since it can actually cause dehydration. Fruits, vegetables, soups, jello, yogurt and other liquid foods all count towards your daily water requirements. For example, several servings of fruits and vegetables can provide as much as 2-3 cups of water daily.

TIP # 48
GREEN TEA FOR WEIGHT LOSS?

According to a recent study reported from London, the daily consumption of green tea was helpful in weight reduction. This weight reduction property is accomplished by a process called ***thermogenesis***. This process is controlled by the sympathetic nervous system, which increases the basal metabolic energy rate, and thus causes fat oxidation. In other words, it causes the burning of fat in the body. There are plant compounds in tea, particularly caffeine and catechins, which work together to increase thermogenesis.

Unlike drugs such as ***ephedrine***, green tea extracts do not increase the heart rate and are not associated with harmful cardiovascular effects. When this process of thermogenesis is increased, the basal metabolic rate increases and fat oxidation occurs. This results in body fat storage being burned.

In a similar study reported in the American Journal of Clinical Nutrition, it was shown that the daily consumption of two cups of green tea increased the basal metabolic rate 4% over a 24-hour period.

It is too early to tell if these studies merit the use of green tea as a weight reduction aid. It is also important to note that many people have sensitivities to caffeine and other plant compounds present in tea, particularly green tea. If you are already a tea drinker and have previously suffered no ill effects, then one to two cups of green tea a day may help with your weight-loss program. Be careful to stay away from health food store extracts or pills that claim to be made from green tea or similar plant extracts. There is no way to find out what other harmful additives these products contain. You should always choose popular brand-name teas for consumption. If you have high blood pressure, heart disease, or diabetes, first check with your physician before trying green tea as a weight reduction aid.

Recent studies indicate that the chemical compounds in green tea can help also to lower your cholesterol. Other studies have shown that green tea can also assist your immune system in fighting off various types of infections. Some researchers go so far as to say that the chemically active substances present in green tea may protect against certain forms of cancer and may help to prevent diabetes. This is starting to sound like the cure-all for all ailments. Remember, most of these studies are preliminary and have yet to be proved. It appears that green tea is a tasty, healthful drink that may help in weight reduction.

In a new study in the September 2004 issue of the Archives of Internal Medicine, it was reported that people who regularly drank green tea had a significant reduction in their blood pressures. The study showed that individuals who consumed 1-2 cups of green tea or oolong tea daily for at least one year reduced their risk of hypertension by at least 65%. Several previous studies reported by Taiwan's National Science Council reported these same blood pressure lowering effects of drinking green tea.

TIP # 49
BREAKFAST FOR YOUR HEART & WAIST

In a recent article in the Archives of Internal Medicine (2004; 164: 370-376), it was reported that *fruit and cereal fiber* might decrease the risk of heart disease. It was thought that the fiber contained in fruit and cereals can lower blood cholesterol and blood pressure, and improve insulin sensitivity, and also make the blood less likely to clot.

Vegetable fiber, however, did not show the same reduced risk of coronary heart disease, which may have been attributed to the failure to distinguish between starchy vegetables (corn and potatoes) and non-starchy vegetables (broccoli and cauliflower). However, due to its high plant nutrient content, vegetable fiber is still extremely important in the reduction of a whole host of degenerative diseases.

This particular study pooled data from ten other studies in the United States and Europe, which included almost 100,000 men and 250,000 women. This study was to determine if dietary fiber actually caused a significant decrease in heart disease. The National Health, Lung and Blood Institute and the Danish Medical Council helped support this study. Over an eight-year follow-up, the risk of coronary heart disease was 10-30% lower for each 10 grams of total fruit or cereal fiber consumed daily. Cereal and fruit for breakfast is truly a heart-healthy meal.

Fiber-rich oatmeal or a cold whole-wheat bran cereal with skim or 1% milk is a great way to start your morning diet. These cereals are nutritious, taste great, and are slow to digest. The high insoluble fiber content of whole grain cereals causes your appetite mechanism to shut down early because of its slow rate of absorption from the intestinal tract. These good tasting whole grain cereal products have also been shown to reduce your craving for high-refined sugar products and fatty foods, such as mid-morning donut or coffee cake snacks.

Oatmeal in particular is also high in soluble fiber, which helps to clean out the fat in your blood vessels by increasing the HDL cholesterol, which sweeps out the bad LDL cholesterol from the bloodstream. Oatmeal for breakfast every day has been recommended by the American Heart Association as a great start for your day to reduce your risk of heart disease while it reduces your waistline.

Cereal can also reduce your risk of developing diabetes. Magnesium also helps to stabilize your blood sugar by preventing the overproduction of insulin by the pancreas. Oatmeal and whole-grain bran-type cereals are good sources of magnesium.

People who eat oatmeal, as well as other whole-grain bran-type cereals daily, have less than one-half the risk of developing obesity and diabetes as non-cereal eaters. High-fiber bran cereals help to regulate insulin production in the morning. This helps to control your appetite and reduce the risk of gaining unwanted pounds. The addition of fruit to your morning cereal, compliments the great taste of the cereal while it boosts your energy level all morning long. Cereal and fruit for breakfast is a really great weight-loss tip!

If you're tired of cereal, then try a non- or low fat yogurt with fresh fruit and low-fat granola or wheat germ. Yogurt with its high calcium and protein content can energize your morning and keeps your hunger at bay until lunch time. The granola or wheat germ will add the necessary fiber to slow your digestion and absorption of your breakfast meal, which in turn helps to keep your appetite satisfied for the entire morning. Yogurt with fruit is a great on-the-go breakfast meal that saves time when you're on your way to work or play.

Another great high protein on-the-go breakfast that satisfies your appetite is a hard-boiled egg and an orange, which are both nutritious and a great tasting, appetite-satisfying breakfast. The high protein and fiber content of an egg and an orange is a healthful breakfast that will help to satisfy your appetite while providing essential nutrients in your diet. Whatever your choice, remember that the combination of lean protein and fiber is another way to keep your appetite satisfied until lunchtime, without the urge for high-calorie, high-fat, mid-morning snacking. You'll pass on the donuts and coffee cake without the least bit of craving.

TIP # 50
DON'T TRY DIET AIDS OR SUPPLEMENTS!

Dietary supplements, herbs, powders, pills, and drinks that contain ephedrine-type compounds known as *ephedra*, or the Chinese herb ma huang, are dangerous to your health. They can cause high blood pressure, strokes, seizures, cardiac arrhythmias, psychotic episodes, and even death. Some states have already banned the sale of these compounds in all consumer products. The American Medical Association has recently recommended that the Food and Drug Administration ban these drugs nationwide because of the serious risk factors associated with them.

The Food and Drug Administration has recently announced plans to ban the sale of all dietary supplements containing ephedra. This is actually the first time the FDA has moved to ban a dietary supplement. Ephedra is contained in a variety of products that make false claims that these products can aid weight-loss, increase energy, and improve athletic performance. The many side effects that are related to ephedra and ephedra-like compounds include dizziness, insomnia, psychosis, heart ailments, increased blood pressure and increased heart rate, dementia, and uterine contractions. There have been many deaths attributed to the use of ephedra, which is contained in these so-called diet pills and supplements.

COMPOUNDS THAT CONTAIN EPHEDRA

Ephedrine
Ma huang or cao ma huang (Chinese ephedra)
Mahuuanggen
Muzei mu huang (Mongolian ephedra)
Natural Ecstasy
Pinellia
Popotillo
Sea grape
Sida cordifolia

Yellow astringent
Yellow horse
Zhong ma huang

The American species of ephedra are often used for teas:
Brigham tea
Desert tea
Mexican tea
Mormon tea
Squaw tea
Teamster's tea

WHY THE FDA IS BANNING EPHEDRA

Many people are currently taking ephedra-containing products to help them lose weight or improve athletic performance. The FDA warns that ephedra-containing substances can have the following adverse reactions in people who use them. These reactions include gastrointestinal symptoms, including diarrhea and cramps; cardiovascular symptoms consisting of palpitations or heart irregularities; neurological conditions such as anxiety, psychosis; hemorrhagic strokes and heart attacks have also been reported. Many of these ephedra or ephedrine compounds also include caffeine in their formulas, which can enhance these possible adverse side effects. These products go by many different names. Some of the popular products found are:

1. Ma huang.
2. Epitonin.
3. Herbal phen-fen is a diet drug, which consists of a combination of ephedra and St. John's Wort.
4. ECA Stack is used by body builders and contains ephedra, caffeine, and aspirin.

BOGUS DIET PILLS

Also, dietary aids that claim they are "fat burners," "carbohydrate busters," "starch blockers" and "muscle builders" are all bogus. They are completely without merit, and, in some cases, they contain a substance called *creatinine*, which can cause kidney damage. Some of these aids can have a laxative effect, and instead of losing weight, you will lose essential vitamins, nutrients, minerals and electrolytes from your body. Some of these bogus diet aids also contain caffeine, which acts as a stimulant and can cause nervousness, palpitations, sweating, diarrhea, anxiety and insomnia. Caffeine does not help to cause weight-loss and is worthless and potentially dangerous as a diet supplement. Many of these products contain a combination of herbs, starch-fillers, and food-dyes that are mixed with a variety of vitamins and minerals, that do nothing but give you indigestion and heartburn.

If a supplement states that you can lose a lot of weight in a short period of time, you can rest assured that it is without merit. There is big money being made in the diet business, especially in diet supplements and so-called weight-loss pills. Diet promoters who make these unrealistic promises are nothing but fast-talking marketing charlatans, who hope that you will buy their products before you realize that they are bogus.

PRESCRIPTION DIET PILLS

The FDA is currently considering taking a popular diet prescription medication off the market because it has amphetamine-like qualities. Amphetamine drugs are extremely dangerous to your health, since they can cause high blood pressure, abnormal heart rhythms, heart attacks and strokes. Let's put it this way: there are no safe diet pills, whether they're over-the-counter pills or those prescribed by a physician. The only way to safely lose weight is to eat less, especially less fat, and to exercise more, particularly walking.

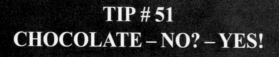

TIP # 51
CHOCOLATE – NO? – YES!

Chocolate has always been the bane of anyone on a diet. Supposedly high in fat and high in calories, it was definitely considered a no-no on any diet plan. There is, however, some good news about chocolate that may have you rethink its value in a healthy diet. Besides tasting good, chocolate may have some healthy redeeming qualities.

First of all, it is packed with flavonoids, which can help to raise your good HDL cholesterol. Secondly, it is rich in antioxidants, which help to combat nasty free radicals, which can cause cell damage. And lastly, chocolate raises those good-feeling chemicals called endorphins, which help to relax and soothe the jangled nerves of the conscientious dieter.

Dark chocolate has more antioxidants than the lighter milk chocolates. The milk in milk chocolate appears to bind the antioxidants, making them unavailable for use in the body. Also, heating chocolate appears to release the antioxidants. So head for the mocha cappuccino, with skim milk, of course, or hot chocolate. There have been some early reports that dark chocolate may even lower blood pressure.

Chocolate is actually good for your heart. Choose dark or bittersweet chocolate, which has three times as many antioxidant compounds (flavonoids) as milk chocolate, and keeps the blood platelets from sticking together, which helps to prevent blood clots from forming.

Calorie-wise, a chocolate-covered small mint patty has only 1.5 grams of total fat and 0.8 grams of saturated fat. A small, thin square of dark chocolate has 3.5 grams of fat and 1.5 grams of saturated fat. A good-tasting treat like chocolate should not be avoided if you are a chocolate lover. Small amounts of dark chocolate taken several times a week will not hinder your diet program, besides tasting great. Actually chocolate is good for weight-loss, since it satisfies your sweet tooth and your brain's hunger mechanism, which prevents you from over-eating. Enjoy!

Several recent studies have shown the heart-protective effects of the antioxidants (cocoa flavonoids), contained in dark chocolate. These antioxidants help to prevent blood clots and inflammation in the arteries that supply blood to the heart. They also help to lower the bad LDL cholesterol and increase the good HDL cholesterol. These recent studies have also shown that the antioxidants found in dark chocolate can reduce blood pressure in patients with high blood pressure. An interesting finding in one study, was that these beneficial cardio-protective effects of dark chocolate, were reduced if the dark chocolate was consumed with milk or milk chocolate. One researcher quipped that, "I guess that means in order to be healthy, you should eat dark chocolate with red wine, therefore combining both of their antioxidant properties." Maybe it's not such a bad idea!

TIP # 52
KEEP YOUR KIDS TRIM & HEALTHY

The number of overweight children has more than tripled in the past 15-20 years. Many studies have indicated that obese children will have shorter life spans than their parents, unless this trend is reversed. If current trends in overeating among children continue, it may well surpass smoking as the primary cause of preventable deaths. Soft drinks are the major source of added sugar for children and adolescents. Many prepared foods, including cakes, cookies, and candies also contain corn-based sweeteners, refined cane sugars, and other sugars. Fast-food restaurants add to the excess number of calories and fat that children consume with their double cheeseburgers topped with fatty sauces, fried chicken and fish sandwiches, and fat-laden French fries.

Teenagers are eating 25% more fat today than they ate 15-20 years ago. A total of 35% of people eat their meals outside the home now, compared to 15% just 10-15 years ago. The tendency is to eat less fruits, vegetables, and whole grains and more high-fat fried foods and soft drinks when eating out, as opposed to eating at home.

Parents should educate their children in healthy eating habits by setting these habits at home and in the restaurant:
1. Discourage second portions of foods at home and downsize portions of food in restaurants. For example, choose a regular-sized hamburger instead of a double cheeseburger with mayo.
2. Substitute salads for French fries, with low-fat or nonfat dressing.
3. Choose regular-sized beverages instead of large-sized beverages.
4. Switch to water, diet sodas, or skim milk.
5. Avoid between-meal snacking.
6. Avoid having high-sugar, high-fat snacks at home (cookies,

cake, and candy).

7. Encourage fruits and vegetables as snacks.
8. Use high-fiber cereals with fruit for breakfast instead of a prepackaged, high-fat, high-calorie breakfast bar or muffin.
9. Limit meats with high fat content.
10. Limit refined carbohydrates (white bread, white rice, baked goods, and most sugar snack foods).
11. Encourage daily exercise. Take your kids for a walk instead of sitting in front of the TV.
12. Let your kids use your stationary bike or treadmill if they can't get out.
13. Encourage children early to develop self-esteem and self-worth by eating healthy and to be proud of their bodies.

MORE TIPS FOR KIDS

1. Eat together as a family as often as possible.
2. Keep healthy snacks in the house; for example, fruits, vegetables, whole-grain breads, peanut butter, sliced turkey breast, sliced low-fat cheeses, and tuna packed in water.
3. Avoid keeping high-fat, high-sugar, high-calorie snack foods; for example, cookies, cakes, chips, candy bars, and high-fat cereal and granola bars.
4. Encourage your children to drink water in place of soft drinks.
5. Limit pancakes and waffles made from refined flour; substitute whole-grain flour products.
6. Never demand that a child "clean his/her plate." Let the child's own appetite determine how much they eat.
7. Never use food as a punishment; for example, "If you don't finish your chores, then there's no dessert."
8. Never use food as a reward; for example, "If you finish your food, then you can have dessert."
9. Avoid eating quickly, which often results in overeating.
10. Avoid eating in front of the TV, which also leads to overeating.

11. Limit the time playing video games, watching TV, or online computer time.
12. Encourage use of the stairs at school and when out shopping in stores, instead of the elevator.
13. Walk or run your pet.
14. Walk to the store for errands.
15. Ride a bike, play sports, and keep active.

Most children, particularly obese children, whose diets consist primarily of junk foods, can develop vitamin and mineral deficiencies. These deficiencies can keep children from reaching their full physical and intellectual potential. This condition has been seen with increasing frequency in the United States, as it has been previously documented in Third World countries, where children develop these deficiencies because of the lack of adequate food available.

Vitamins and minerals are essential micronutrients that are needed by the body in small amounts in order to provide proper nutrition for growth and development. Some nutrient deficiencies are:

1. Iron deficiency-impaired intellectual development in young children.
2. Zinc deficiency can result in stunted growth, diarrhea, and lung problems.
3. Vitamin A deficiency lowers a child's immunity level and makes them more susceptible to viral and bacterial infections.
4. Iodine deficiency during pregnancy and in infants and young children can result in mental impairment.
5. B-complex deficiencies can result in a variety of neurological and blood disorders.

Fortunately, vitamin and mineral supplements are inexpensive and are readily available in the United States. All children, particularly those who are overweight and whose diets are deficient in these micronutrients, should take a multivitamin/mineral supplement daily.

Other groups of people are also likely to lack the nutrients found in multivitamin/mineral pills. These groups are defined as low-calorie dieters, obese adults, teenagers with poor eating habits, pregnant women, and senior citizens with poor diets. A daily vitamin and mineral supplement can lessen the incidence of infections and reduce the risk of heart disease, osteoporosis, cancer, and macular degeneration of the eyes.

TIP # 53
KEEP A FOOD AND EXERCISE DIARY

Before you start any diet or exercise plan, get a small notebook and record the following:

1. The time you eat each meal.
2. What you ate and drank at each meal. Be specific, including amounts.
3. Estimate portion sizes.
    a. Your fist size is about one-half cup of pasta, rice, or vegetables.
    b. Your palm size is about 3-4 ounces of protein.
4. Where were you when you ate? At home, at work, at a party, etc.
5. Were you hungry?
6. Were you stressed, relaxed, bored, angry, or guilty?
7. Record physical activity for that day.
8. Weigh yourself only one time a week.

After a week or two, look back over your entries to see what type of eater you are. This is a self-test, with no grades and no wrong answers:

1. Are you eating two, three or four meals a day?
2. Do you snack regularly?
3. How long do you go between meals or snacks?
4. Are you eating because you are hungry or bored, angry or guilty?
5. Do certain emotions trigger binge snack-food eating?
6. Are you eating healthy foods, such as fruits, vegetables, lean protein, and whole-grain products?
7. Are you eating junk foods that are high in fat and calories?
8. How many calories are you eating daily, and how much fat and sugar do you consume?
9. Were you hungry when you ate, or did you just eat because you thought it was time to eat?

   10. Are you getting any exercise at all?

   11. Are you eating while watching TV or at the computer?

   12. Do you eat late at night, just before bedtime?

Now, after you've analyzed your self-test, you can start to adjust your eating and exercise habits slowly, one step at a time:

1. Set small steps for yourself that you can easily achieve. For example, add more fruits and less high-calorie, high-fat foods next week.

2. Don't concentrate on trying to lose 15 pounds in the next month.

3. The following week, add more vegetables to your meals and decrease the amount of starchy vegetables like corn and white potatoes.

4. The following week, substitute whole-grain cereals and breads for refined grains, like white rice, white bread, and baked goods.

5. Start to analyze when you eat, and try to eat your meals at regular times each day and in the same place.

6. Eat only at the kitchen table, not in front of the TV, computer, or on the phone.

7. Eat only until you are not hungry any longer. Don't wait until you're full.

8. Have a piece of fruit for a midmorning or midafternoon snack.

9. Eat a nonfat yogurt at bedtime to satisfy your sweet tooth.

10. There are even low-fat, low-calorie TV dinners that you don't have to bother preparing.

11. It is not only what you eat, but how many calories you consume. So be conscious of the total calorie content of your meals.

12. Control portion sizes. Eat only one-half of a restaurant meal and take the other half home for tomorrow.

13. Start a regular exercise program by walking 15 minutes a day for the first two weeks.

14. Then walk 20 minutes a day for two weeks.

15. Then begin walking 30 minutes a day for two weeks.

16. It is easy to take walking breaks during lunch, after dinner, or in the morning, whenever it fits conveniently into your schedule.

This diary is just the starting point to see what type of an eater you are. It's easy to modify your eating habits by just taking small steps each week to change from poor eating habits to good ones. Rome wasn't built in a day, and neither were you. Once you start to see results, in particular a drop in pants or dress size, you will know that healthy eating and a healthy, trim body go hand in hand.

TIP # 54
DON'T BE A YO-YO DIETER

The Framingham Heart Study, which has followed more than 5,000 people for almost 40 years, recently indicated a health hazard for chronic dieters. People who lost 10% of their body weight had an almost 20% reduction in the incidence of heart disease. So what's the problem? These same dieters who gained back the 10% of their body weight, *raised their heart disease risk by almost 30%.* So if you weighed 160 pounds and lost 10% or 16 pounds, you decreased your heart disease risk by 20%. But if you gained back those 16 pounds, you increased your risk of heart attack by 30%, an overall net gain of 10%, and you still weight the same 160 pounds. *Sounds scary to me, folks!* How many times have you heard the old saying that "I've lost enough weight over the years to equal two or three whole persons, and I've gained every bit of it back?" *Yo-yo dieting or weight-cycling* makes it harder to permanently lose weight and is much more dangerous to your health.

Experts in the fields of physiology, biochemistry, psychology, nutrition, and medicine have come up with the following startling findings about yo-yo dieting:

1.   The weight-loss/weight-gain cycle actually *increases your desire for fatty foods*. Animal research studies at Yale University showed that rats which had lost weight rapidly on low-calorie diets always chose more fat in their diets when given a choice between fat, protein, and carbohydrates. These rats always put on more weight than when they started, and in a much shorter time than it had taken them to lose the weight.

2.   Yo-yo dieters *increase the percentage of body fat* to lean body tissue with repeated bouts of weight gain and weight-loss. Women who lose weight rapidly on a low-carbohydrate, high-protein diet can lose a significant amount of muscle tissue. If the weight is regained again, they usually regain more fat and less muscle because it is easier for the body to gain fat than it is to rebuild muscle tissue.

3. *Body fat gets redistributed in the abdomen* from the thighs, buttocks, and hips after weight cycling. Medical research has definitely shown that fat deposits above the waist increase the risk of heart disease and diabetes, not to mention an unsightly paunch.

4. When you lose weight by cutting calories, your basal metabolic rate (BMR) slows down, because it is the body's defense mechanism against starvation. The body can't tell the difference between starvation and low-calorie dieting; consequently, your body is trying to conserve energy by burning fewer calories. This is the reason it becomes harder to lose weight after a week or two, even though you are eating exactly the same amount of calories as you did when you first started your diet. This slowdown in the basal metabolic rate (BMR) persists, even after the diet is over, and accounts for the rapid-rebound, excessive weight gain that always happens to the dieter when she or he goes off the diet. This slowdown in metabolic rate can occur even after a single attempt at dieting. However, the repeated effects of weight-cycling diets can affect the basal metabolic rate (BMR) much more, making additional weight-loss almost impossible and rebound weight gain almost inevitable. The yo-yo dieter is often heard to say – "I'm heavier now than I was before I started this damn diet."

5. An enzyme called *lipoprotein lipase* (LPL) becomes more active when you cut calories. This enzyme controls the amount of fat that is stored in your body's fat cells. Dieting, therefore, makes the body more efficient at storing fat, which is exactly the opposite of what a dieter wants. As you reduce your calorie intake, the enzyme LPL starts to activate the fat-storing process. This is another defense mechanism that the body uses to prevent starvation. Remember, the enzyme LPL doesn't know that you are dieting; it thinks that you are starving to death.

6. Women dieters who have lost a substantial amount of weight were compared to women of normal weight. After they lost weight, the previously obese women needed surprisingly fewer calories to maintain their weight than the normal-weight women. Who said dieting was fair?

7.   Female dieters who exhibited repeated cycles of weight gain and weight-loss showed an increased risk of sudden death from heart attacks, according to a recent medical report. This study followed 1,500 women over a period of 25 years, who had engaged in cyclic-dieting.

Yo-yo diets may also actually harm the immune system. In a new study reported in the June 2004 issue of the American Dietetic Association, women who had a history of repeatedly losing and regaining weight had weaker immune systems than women who did not engage in yo-yo dieting. Those women who reported losing and regaining weight more than five times over a period of years, were found to have 1/3 lower natural killer cells in the blood stream, which are essential for the body's immune system to kill viruses and bacteria. This is yet another reason to avoid fad diets, particularly low-carb diets, which are notorious for rebound weight gain. A sensible approach to dieting therefore is a lifestyle change that incorporates healthy eating habits combined with a regular exercise program of walking.

TIP # 55
FIGHT REBOUND WEIGHT GAIN

So, what's the answer to preventing rebound weight gain?

We know that losing weight lowers blood pressure, reduces the risk of heart disease, lowers blood cholesterol and triglycerides, and increases the HDL ("good" cholesterol). The answer is that dieting alone is not the best way to lose and maintain weight. The following is a list of the reasons why *walking, combined with a high-fiber, low-fat diet plan, is the safest and most effective method* to lose and maintain normal body weight:

1. Exercise, particularly walking, is the real answer to preventing the weight-loss/weight gain cycle from occurring. Walking makes it less likely you'll gain the weight back again because you lose more fat and less muscle tissue with exercise. Also, walking prevents the slowdown in basal metabolic rate that always occurs with a yo-yo diet. Actually, walking slightly increases the BMR, which helps to burn calories at a faster rate. Walking also reduces the production of the enzyme lipoprotein lipase (LPL), which, in turn, decreases the amount of fat stored in the fat cells.

2. Walking also regulates the brain's appetite controller, the appestat. The more you walk, the more you decrease the appestat's hunger mechanism. Inactivity, on the other hand, stimulates the appetite control mechanism to make you hungry.

3. Walking, by increasing the aerobic metabolism of the body, redirects the stomach's blood supply to the exercising muscles, which, in turn, decreases your appetite.

4. And finally, walking encourages the body to burn fat rather than carbohydrates. This enables the body's blood sugar to stay at a relatively constant normal level. When the brain's blood sugar is normal, we are not hungry. Both strenuous exercise and low-

calorie dieting, however, burn carbohydrates rather than fats, causing a sharp drop in the blood sugar. When the brain's blood sugar drops, as it does in very low calorie diets or strenuous exercises, then we feel hungry in order to counteract this low blood sugar. A high-fiber, low-fat, lean protein diet also controls the body's appetite center, making overeating high-fat calories next to impossible.

5. Most importantly, stay away from any diet that restricts one type of food group, like low carbohydrate diets. Not only are these diets unhealthy, but also once they're stopped as they will invariably be, because of boredom or illness, then rebound weight gain packs on the pounds faster than a speeding bullet.

6. And lastly, in order to really prevent rebound weight gain, stick with a healthy, good tasting diet consisting of fruits, vegetables, whole grain products, and lean protein. Even when this type of diet is bent slightly in favor of an occasional sweet treat, rebound weight gain does not occur. This is the type of diet that can last you for a lifetime and will also make that lifetime last.

TIP # 56
SMALL FREQUENT MEALS
BURN FAT FASTER

After a meal, the pancreas (an endocrine gland located behind your stomach) produces a hormone called insulin, which is released into the bloodstream. A meal that is high in fat or sugar causes the pancreas to release a lot more insulin than does a meal which is high in complex carbohydrates. Likewise, a larger meal causes more insulin to be released than a smaller meal.

One of insulin's functions is to regulate the level of sugar in the blood by burning carbohydrates and conserving stores of body fat from the body's fat cells, where it could be burned as fuel for energy. As you can see then, this is not a good thing, because the fat stays in the fat cells, and you stay fat while you're trying to diet. Also, high levels of insulin promote the absorption of dietary fat into the body's fat cells. In other words, the higher the level of insulin, the more fat that is absorbed into your fat cells and the less fat that can get out of the cells.

More frequent, smaller meals, on the other hand, tend to keep the pancreas from producing excess amounts of insulin. This results in more dietary fat being burned as fuel, which results in less fat being stored in the fat cells. Also, less insulin encourages the breakdown of fat already in your fat cells, to be released into the blood to be used as an additional fuel for energy.

In other words, small, frequent complex-carbohydrate meals produce steady, lower levels of insulin being released into the bloodstream than does eating larger, high-fat, high-sugar meals. Therefore, small, frequent complex-carbohydrate meals result in more fat being burned as a fuel and less fat being stored as fat deposits. As an added benefit of eating small, frequent complex-carbohydrate meals, you actually produce a decrease in your appetite. This is due to the fact that, as you burn more fat, you are actually using up calories, instead of storing calories.

TIP # 57
DIET FALLACIES

1. **Calories don't count. False!** This is the first of the many fallacies that people use in the weight-loss business. On the contrary, calories do count in a weight-gain, weight-loss program. In order to lose a pound of fat, you must reduce your intake by 3,500 calories. However, in a low-fat, moderate lean protein and moderate complex carbohydrate diet there is no need to count calories, since by nature this is a low calorie diet.

2. **A crash diet** is an excellent way to begin a weight-loss program. **False!** This is probably the worst way to begin a diet program, since most crash diets, which are usually low in carbohydrates, produce rapid fluid loss. This fluid loss has nothing to do with the amount of liquid that we drink, and it is only reflecting a change in the body's ability to hold fluid. The fallacy is that fat is not coming off in this type of program and, in fact, protein can be lost during a crash diet, which may be harmful to the kidneys. When these diets are abandoned, weight is gained rapidly, usually in the form of fat, and the dieter may wind up with more fat than when he or she started.

3. **Exercise is unimportant** in weight reduction and control. **False!** Nothing can be further from the truth. Regular physical exercise and activity is the key point in a long-term weight reduction and weight maintenance program. Exercise not only burns calories, but also has an appetite-regulating effect on the brain's appetite control mechanism. Exercise also favorably affects the metabolism by lowering blood pressure, blood cholesterol, blood sugar, and, in general, contributing to good health.

4. **Eating more in the morning** will put on less weight than eating food in the evening. **False!** The body does not

distinguish between time of day and calories consumed. It is the total amount of calories that you consume daily that determines your weight.

5. **Certain foods can burn up calories,** such as grapefruit. **False!** This is entirely erroneous. The digestion of food does consume some energy in the process of digestion, but there is no food that expends enough energy during digestion to promote weight-loss.

6. **It is better to smoke than to be fat. False!** The initial weight gained from decreasing or stopping smoking can always be lost by a diet and exercise program; however, the permanent lung, heart, and artery damage done by smoking can never be undone.

7. **Toasting bread reduces its calorie count. False!** Toasting only changes the bread's texture and taste, but does not burn away calories.

8. **It does not make any difference whether you eat slowly or quickly, as far as appetite or weight gain are concerned. False!** Eating a meal slowly and chewing the food thoroughly gives the body's metabolism a chance to regulate and reduce its appetite-regulating center in the brain. This subsequently can reduce the appetite and make you more satisfied with less food. Eating rapidly does not cause overweight; however, since many overweight people tend to eat rapidly and do not give the appetite suppressing mechanism time to work, they eat more.

9. **Since meat is high in protein, it does not cause weight gain. False!** Protein, no matter what the source, contains 4 calories per gram. Carbohydrate also contains 4 calories per gram. Fat, however, contains 9 calories per gram, more than twice as many calories as a gram of protein or carbohydrate. Since any excessive calories above the body's basic metabolic requirements results in an increased storage of fat, eating meat not only can cause weight gain, but can cause a greater proportion of fat being deposited in the body because of its high fat content.

Therefore, meat not only gives 4 calories per gram for its protein content, but it also gives 9 calories per gram for its fat content. Therefore, the greater the percentage of fat in the meat, the higher the caloric value.

10.   **As long as you take a vitamin supplement every day, it doesn't matter what foods you eat or drink. False!** Vitamin supplements will not provide all the daily requirements of protein, carbohydrates, minerals, amino acids, and essential fatty acids that the body needs. This is a widespread misconception about nutrition and dieting. Many complications have been noted by people on very low-calorie diets combined with protein-vitamin supplements, because of the inability of the body's metabolism, particularly the kidneys and liver, to adjust to this type of diet.

11.   **If I skip breakfast and lunch, and just eat a large supper, I will lose weight. False!** No matter when the calories are consumed in a given 24-hour period, the total end result is the same. The basic formula is: Calories consumed vs. calories expended. Whether you eat 400 calories three times a day or 1,200 calories at one meal, the body does not know the difference. In addition, skipping meals is not a healthful way to embark on a diet program, since the appetite becomes overstimulated late in the day, and you not only eat a large dinner, but you also eat continuous snacks through the evening.

12.   **If I eat or snack at bedtime, the food will not be digested properly and I will gain weight. False!** Again, the same principle exists, as to the total calories consumed in any 24-hour period vs. the total calories expended. This is the basic formula needed for either weight gain, weight-loss, or weight maintenance. Eating at bedtime will not put any more weight on than eating at any other time of day or night. Some people, however, may develop indigestion when they eat immediately before bedtime.

TIP # 58
LOSE WEIGHT WITH POWER FOODS

MUSHROOMS

Many types of mushrooms contain the amino acid *glutamic acid*, which boosts the immune system and helps to fight various types of infections. By helping to improve the body's immune system, mushrooms have also been known to fight certain forms of cancer and autoimmune diseases, such as rheumatoid arthritis, lupus, and other collagen diseases. Mushrooms are also rich in potassium and vitamin C, which help to keep blood pressure normal.

Portobello and white mushrooms have a high content of certain nutrients and minerals, particularly selenium, which may help to reduce the risk of prostate and breast cancer. When selenium is combined with the vitamin E present in mushrooms, it helps to prevent nasty free radicals from damaging the body's normal cells, thus slowing the aging process.

Shiitake mushrooms also contain many plant nutrients, in particular lentinan and eritadenine, which help to improve the immune system and assist in lowering blood cholesterol. These phyto-nutrients have also been shown to reduce the risk of heart disease and certain forms of cancer.

All mushrooms are low in calories and are fat-free, making them excellent staples in a weight-loss program. They are excellent flavor enhancers for a variety of foods. Mushrooms are not only good for you, but they are great for your weight-loss program.

GRAPEFRUIT

Grapefruit contains high levels of potassium, vitamin C, beta-carotene, and the antioxidant lycopene, which has been shown to reduce the risk of both breast and prostate cancers. Grapefruits also contain bioflavonoids, which appear to protect against heart disease. They also contain phyto-nutrients, which include *phenolic acid*, which can block nitrosamines, which are cancer-causing chemicals found in many smoked foods.

Grapefruits are a great addition to any weight-reduction program, since they are low in calories and high in fiber. The only precaution is that patients who are on cholesterol-lowering drugs called statins should be careful about drinking grapefruit juice with these medications. Grapefruit juice appears to slow the natural breakdown of these drugs in the bloodstream, causing higher than expected levels of these medications to stay active in the blood for longer periods of time. It is important for any patient on statin medication to check with his or her doctor before combining grapefruit with these cholesterol-lowering drugs.

PIZZA

According to the Harvard School of Public Health, tomato sauce contains an antioxidant called *lycopene*, which has been proven to reduce the risk of heart disease and certain forms of cancer, including breast and prostate cancer. A study of over 5,000 people showed that those who ate pizza one to two times per week decreased their risk of different forms of cancer by over 50%.

Tomato sauce has more lycopene than just ordinary tomatoes, since it is thought to be the heating process of tomatoes that releases the healthy lycopene into the tomato sauce. Pizza's tomato sauce is an excellent way to reduce your risk of heart disease and certain forms of cancer.

Pizza is also more filling than many foods, causing you to eat fewer calories and become appetite-satisfied earlier. You can bump up the lycopene content and decrease the calorie content of pizza by ordering your pizza with light or no cheese, and extra tomato sauce. A tomato pie or pizza is a great way to lose weight and improve your health. If you do order a regular pizza, make sure you use several napkins to blot up the extra fat before eating. You can reduce the total calorie content of each piece of pizza by more than 25% by using this fat-blotting napkin method.

OLIVE OIL AND OLIVES

Olive oil and olives contain heart-healthy monounsaturated fats. These friendly fats help to reduce your appetite by satisfying your body's craving for high-refined sugars and empty calories. Olives and olive oil are both low in saturated fats, and by only eating small amounts of these monounsaturated fats, your appetite is quickly satisfied and fewer calories are consumed. These healthy fats fill you up fast and satisfy your appetite quickly.

Monounsaturated fats present in olive oil, olives, nuts, and avocados have been shown to reduce both blood pressure and blood cholesterol. These heart-healthy fats are the staples of many Mediterranean countries, which have considerably less obesity and heart disease than does the United States.

ONIONS AND GARLIC

These two vegetables contain plant nutrients that break down fat globules from food in the intestinal tract, preventing this fat from being absorbed into the body. Less fat absorbed means less fat stored in your fat cells, which translates into less weight gained.

Onions contain a phytonutrient called *quercetin*, which has been shown to keep blood from clotting by reducing the stickiness of the blood platelets. This helps to reduce the risk of heart attacks and strokes.

Garlic contains several phyto-nutrients that also help to reduce the incidence of heart disease and have been shown to inactivate certain viruses that cause intestinal and respiratory illnesses.

FISH

Fish are low in calories, low in fat, and high in protein, which makes them ideal for any real weight-loss plan. Even shellfish with its higher content of cholesterol is still an important fat-burning food in your diet program. The low saturated fat content of shellfish offsets any cholesterol that these products may contain.

The high protein content in fish acts as the fat-burner, since the protein increases your basal metabolic rate. Fat is subsequently burned more quickly and weight-loss becomes quick and easy. Low mercury-containing fish eaten three times a week has been proven to help dieters lose weight easily and help to keep that weight off permanently. Fish also contain omega-3 fatty acids that help to reduce your risk of heart disease, strokes, cancer, and neurological disorders, such as Alzheimer's disease.

The omega-3 fatty acids in fish have been shown to lower blood cholesterol and to reduce the incidence of certain forms of cancer. The omega-3 fats appear to block the action of certain genes, which are involved in the formation of both colon and breast cancer. Salmon, sardines, trout, and herring are particularly high in omega fats, Despite the reports that farmed salmon may contain more chemicals than wild salmon, the American Institute for Cancer Research says that the benefits of eating fish, whether farmed or wild, outweighs the risks.

TIP # 59
REALLY GREAT DIET TIPS

1. **Eat more slowly with each meal.** This involves taking smaller, less frequent bites and chewing each mouthful for a longer period of time. Pause between each section of the meal.
2. If you are still hungry when you are finished with your first portion, **wait at least 15 minutes** to see whether or not you really want another portion. In most cases, your appestat (the brain appetite control mechanism) will be more than satisfied at the end of that period of time, and you will not need a second helping.
3. Also restrict your meals to one, or perhaps two, locations in your home for eating. If you have no regular place to eat, then you will find that you are eating in every room; however, when food is restricted to **one main dining area**, there will be fewer tendencies to snack during the day.
4. Make sure you **leave the table** as soon as you are finished eating and spend **less time in the kitchen** or areas that have a tendency to remind one of eating.
5. Make sure that you do not place **serving dishes** on the table during a meal, for there will be more of a tendency to take second and third helpings. Be sure that you **do not leave food out** where you can repeatedly see it during the day.
6. Never go to the market on an empty stomach; you will buy snack foods (carbohydrates cravings). Also, make it a point not to eat while watching **television** or **reading**, since you will eat more while not concentrating on your meal.
7. Remember not to start a weight reduction program just prior to the **holiday season** or before **vacation time**, since these are the most unsuccessful times to begin this type of project.
8. **Fried foods** should be avoided, since, even though you drain excess fat away, fried foods still retain a large percentage of fat,

which adds to the calories. **Boiling, broiling, baking, or steaming** are the best techniques for preparing foods.

9. **Fat on poultry and meat:** Always trim away visible fat from meat and fowl before cooking, and remove visible fat at the table when eating. The skin of the chicken contains 25% of the fat content of the chicken and will add tremendously to the calories. Canned fishes, such as tuna and salmon, should be packed in water or have the oils drained away.

10. **Hot foods,** such as soups, and foods that require a lot of **chewing** will leave you with a greater feeling of satisfaction because they take a longer time to swallow and absorb. Make sure you **leave the table** as soon as you finish eating.

11. Eat salad **greens** and **vegetables** before the main course, since these will take the edge off your hunger for higher calorie meat, poultry, and fish portions. The best salad dressing is none. Salad dressings are high in fats and calories. Use calorie-free herbs, spices, lemon, vinegar, or occasionally a small amount (1 tsp.) nonfat, low-calorie dressing. **Restaurant tip:** Dip your fork in a side cup of salad dressing every 3-4 mouthfuls of salad, and you'll enjoy the taste without the extra calories.

12. **Teflon-coated pans** and the new nonfat **edible spray-on coatings**, which are made of vegetable oil, will help reduce the amount of caloric fat that you consume. Although **margarine** is lower in saturated fats than butter, it is still 100% fat, and has almost as many calories as butter, not to mention the bad fats (trans fats).

13. **Alcohol:** Excessive alcohol is one of the most serious hazards in any diet program, whether it is dining out or at home. The additional calories which are consumed in the American diet from alcohol, have a tendency to cause and maintain overweight problems. Alcohol has more calories (7 calories per gram) than most foods on a weight basis. Try to substitute club soda with a twist of lemon, or mineral water, for drinks. Limit your alcohol intake to 4 oz. of red wine or 12 oz. of light beer three times per week.

VII.
SECRET
GET-SLIM
TIPS

TIP # 60
BEAT FOOD CRAVINGS

Food cravings may have a **physiological** as well as an **emotional** component, according to many researchers. Those eating binges or cravings for ice cream, pizza, and hoagies may not necessarily begin in the stomach.

CARBOHYDRATE CRAVINGS for sweets, cakes, pretzels, potato chips, and crackers may be caused *by low blood sugar.* This condition can occur when you have not eaten for several hours or because of emotional frustration, and has been noted to be present prior to the menstrual period because of hormonal fluctuations. Complex carbohydrates like fruits, vegetables, and whole-grain cereals can reduce the craving for refined carbohydrates. High-protein, non-fat milk and low-fat (skim milk) cheese can also cut this craving.

SALT CRAVINGS, such as pickles, potato chips, and olives, can result from a *salt depletion* caused by excessive perspiration, or a *stress condition*, which results in the stimulation of the adrenal glands. Salt cravings can be reduced by substituting lemon juice and herbs, and adding fresh fruit (orange, grapefruit, banana, cantaloupe, tomatoes, or strawberries) to the diet that has a high vitamin C content, which can reduce the craving for salt.

CAFFEINE is present in coffee, tea and cola drinks. Cocoa and chocolate contain theobromine (a caffeine-type substance). Many people are actually *addicted* both physiologically and metabolically to caffeine and will suffer emotional *withdrawal symptoms*, which include headache, fatigue, nausea, irritability, and even a craving for sugar. To reduce this addiction, you have to gradually reduce the caffeine in your diet by substituting *non-caffeine* drinks, such as decaffeinated coffee, herbal teas, clear diet sodas other than colas, and mineral water or club soda.

EMOTIONS AND FOOD CRAVINGS

People who are anxious or stressed out have a tendency to crave sweets and high-calorie foods. Anxiety and stress cause your adrenal glands and pituitary gland to produce certain hormones that stimulate your brain's hunger mechanism to crave refined sugars and carbohydrates (cakes, pies, doughnuts, and candy bars). These quick-fix carbs tend to quell anxiety temporarily by the sudden rise in blood sugar, which causes a feeling of calm. However, with the rapid rise in blood sugar comes a rapid spike in insulin and a more rapid drop in blood sugar, causing anxiety to quickly return.

You can beat anxiety and stress food cravings by eating low-calorie, crunchy foods, such as apples, celery, carrot sticks, or low-fat pretzels (whole-wheat or sourdough). The crunch factor gives your stress-induced anxiety time to cool down without causing a rapid rise in your blood sugar. The actual process of chewing causes your facial and neck muscles to relax, which, in turn, relieves stress and tension.

If you are depressed or sad, your first inclination is also to head for the sweet bar instead of the salad bar. The quick-fix of sugar raises the blood sugar, which, in turn, spikes the pancreas's insulin production. High levels of insulin in the blood increase the production of *serotonin*, which improves your emotional mood. You feel more relaxed and mellow, which is actually how antidepressant drugs work, by increasing your brain's serotonin levels. Unfortunately, serotonin levels plummet after insulin levels drop, and the feeling of sadness and depression quickly returns. To combat this feeling, you can boost your serotonin levels for longer periods of time by eating fruits when you are feeling down. Fruits only gradually increase the level of blood sugar because fruit sugar, or fructose, is slowly absorbed. Insulin levels then become graduated, causing a sustained, long-lived blood and brain serotonin levels.

People who eat because they are bored or just plain tired often eat high-calorie, refined sugar carbohydrate snacks, like cakes and candies, which are readily available and easy to buy or consume. A mocha caffeinated latte may taste good, but the caffeine and sugar interfere with the production of endorphins and serotonin. Instead of feeling relaxed and calm, you will feel edgy and wired. Nuts, particularly almonds and walnuts, are great boredom snacks, since they provide omega-3 fatty acids that can relieve the feelings of fatigue and boredom. Combined with raisins, nuts make the ideal feel-good, energy-boosting snack.

People who are unhappy or in a bad mood often turn to high-fat, high-carbohydrate foods, like pizza or cheese steaks smothered in onions. These foods contain protein and fat, both of which help to produce good-feeling endorphins. On the other hand, they also produce tons of fat and calories, which help to destroy any well-intentioned diet plan. To cause an increase in the production of endorphins, substitute high-fiber, whole-grain cereals and breads for the refined carbs, and substitute lean protein, low-fat cheeses, yogurt, turkey, chicken, and fish for the extra-unwanted fat calories. These complex carbohydrates and high-protein foods produce both endorphins and serotonin to keep your mood happy and euphoric. Boost your mood with less fat and less calories. Be happy!

TIP # 61
WHY WOMEN GAIN WEIGHT EASILY

Unfortunately, women gain weight easier and faster than men, which is partially due to a woman's slower metabolism. Men have more muscle mass and burn fat at a faster rate than women. So it is important that women exercise regularly in order to burn calories and to increase their metabolic rates. Women, however, have a distinct advantage over men in that they naturally have more sustained endurance when they exercise. So that women who engage in a regular sustained aerobic exercise program burn more fat calories than men who do strenuous exercises for short periods of time, since quick bursts of energy burn primarily carbohydrates rather than fat. Therefore, sustained aerobic exercise helps women increase their metabolic rates during exercise and also at rest.

It also takes longer for a woman to digest food than it does for a man. Because of the slower production of certain digestive enzymes, women metabolize fat and a number of medications, including alcohol, at a slower rate than men. Fat in a woman's diet, therefore, causes her to gain weight easily because of this inability to digest and metabolize fat quickly.

So it's no wonder that fat in a woman's diet is just about the worst thing that she can have in order to lose weight and stay healthy. Fat contains 9 calories per gram, and combined with a women's slower rate of metabolism, considerably more fat is stored in her fat cells.

Increasing lean protein and complex carbohydrates in a woman's diet and reducing saturated fats makes it much easier for her to digest and absorb food for the maximum weight-loss effect.

Low carbohydrate diets, which are essentially high fat diets, make it even more difficult for women to lose weight, and, in particular, to keep the weight off. These diets don't work and they are very toxic to their bodies. Initial weight-loss is always followed by marked rebound weight gain.

TIP # 62
SECRET WEIGHT-LOSS FORMULA
FOR WOMEN

SECRET FORMULA PART #1:
20 GRAMS OF TOTAL FAT

- Fat contains 9 calories per gram whereas both carbohydrate and protein contain only 4 calories per gram.
- Excess fat in the diet causes heart disease, diabetes, vascular disease and breast and uterine cancer.
- Less fat in the diet results in more storage fat being burned as fuel so both you and your fat cells become nice and thin.
- 1 pound of body fat contains 3,500 calories, which makes it very easy to gain weight when you eat fat, since fat contains more than twice the number of calories as carbohydrate and protein.
- Fat is the number 1 killer of both your heart and your figure.
- Eat no more than 20 grams of total fat calories daily to lose weight.
- Consult a chart for the total grams of fat in various foods and keep a record of what you eat.
- To maintain your ideal weight, eat no more than 25 grams of fat daily.

SECRET FORMULA PART #2:
20 GRAMS OF DIETARY FIBER

- Fiber helps you to lose weight because of the slower emptying of the stomach and makes you feel full earlier.
- Fiber contains fewer calories for its large volume so that it fills you up without filling you out.

- Fiber has a high bulk ratio, which makes your hunger center satisfied more quickly.
- Fiber has the ability to absorb lots of water and therefore regulates the progression of food through the digestive system.
- Fiber helps to lower blood cholesterol and also decreases the risk of heart disease, hypertension and stroke.
- Fiber helps to keep the digestive system healthy.
- Fruits, vegetables and whole grains are not only high in fiber but also contain many nutrients and antioxidants.
- To lose weight, eat at least 20 grams of dietary fiber daily.
- Consult a chart for the total grams of fiber in various foods and keep a record of what you eat.
- To maintain your ideal weight, eat no less than 15 grams of dietary fiber daily.

SECRET FORMULA PART # 3:
20 MINUTES WALKING DAILY

- Walking is the ideal aerobic exercise for good health, fitness and weight-loss without the dangers of strenuous exercise.
- Walking burns approximately 350 calories per hour, so you can lose 1 pound of body fat for every 10 hours you walk.
- Strenuous exercise burns primarily carbohydrates to produce energy and does very little to help you to lose weight.
- As strenuous exercise burns carbohydrates it produces a drop in blood sugar, which actually increases your appetite.
- Slow, continuous, moderate activity like walking burns primarily fat stored in the body and is the best exercise for sustained weight-loss. You lose more fat and less muscle.
- Walking increases the body's metabolic rate, which helps to burn calories at a faster rate.

- Walking as an aerobic exercise re-directs blood away from the stomach to the exercising muscles and decreases appetite.
- Walking regulates the brain's appetite center. Walking before a meal decreases the appetite.
- Walking has the added benefit of decreasing the risk of heart disease, hypertension, stroke and certain forms of cancer.
- A 20-minute brisk walk daily will burn enough calories to help you lose weight quickly. 10-minutes twice a day is just as good.
- Once you've reached your ideal weight, take a day off and rest.

TIP # 63
A REALLY EASY WEIGHT- LOSS TIP

There is an easy way to figure out how many calories you are eating every day to maintain your current weight. Multiply your current weight by 12, which will equal the number of calories needed daily to maintain your current weight.

Example: If you weigh 150 pounds, multiply that by 12, which will equal 1,800 calories. 1,800 calories then is the number of calories that you need every day to maintain your 150 pounds.

Or, for example, if you weigh 125 pounds, then multiply 125 x 12 = 1,500 calories, which means that a 125-pound person only needs 1,500 calories a day to maintain his or her 125-pound weight.

One easy technique for losing weight is to reduce your calorie intake by 300 calories per day, and increase your activity level by 200 calories per day. This is a total of 500 calories lost per day. Since 3,500 calories equal one pound, you will be able to lose one pound per week, with little or no effort. That calculation is as follows: You are taking in 300 less calories per day and burning up 200 calories per day with activities such as walking, which equals 500 calories lost per day, x 7 days per week = 3,500 calories, which means you have lost one pound in one week.

You can also reduce your calorie intake by 500 calories per day with no increase in your activity level and still lose a pound a week (500 calories reduced from diet x 7 days = 3,500 calories or one pound weight-loss). Just think of the weight-loss possibilities by decreasing the calorie intake every day and increasing your activity level by more than a total of 500 calories per day.

Slow and steady weight-loss is the safest and most effective way to lose weight and to maintain that weight-loss. Also, slow and steady weight- loss helps to condition you to make permanent changes in your eating habits, which, in effect, is what we are striving to do for permanent weight-loss. Regular exercise also conditions your body to expect regular physical activity every day for a feeling of well-being. Sounds simple? It certainly is!

TIP # 64
ARE YOU REALLY OVERWEIGHT?

Obesity is actually an epidemic in the United States. More than 60% of adults are overweight, and 30% of these overweight people are actually considered obese. The increased risks with obesity are heart disease, diabetes, strokes, arthritis, and various forms of cancer. What's the reason for this epidemic? *People in the United States are eating more and exercising less.*

In restaurants, portion sizes are getting larger. Soft drinks have ballooned in size from 8 ounces to 24 ounces; hamburgers, cheeseburgers, and French fries sold at fast-food chains are three to four times larger than they were ten years ago.

We are burning fewer calories every day due to the lack of exercise. With the so-called energy-saving devices, such as TVs with their remotes, golf carts, riding lawnmowers, bank and fast-food windows, and eight-hour desk jobs, Americans are burning fewer calories than ever. Only one out of every four to five of us gets at least 20-30 minutes of exercise three times per week, and the rest of us get little or no exercise at all. So how do you tell if you are overweight or actually obese? There is a very complicated measurement known as the **Body Mass Index**, or BMI, that can tell you the answer. Needless to say, you have to consult a chart to find out the answer, unless you are a whiz at algebra. The basic premise, however, is that depending on your height (in inches) and your weight (in pounds), if your BMI is between 25-30, you are overweight. If your BMI is greater than 30, you are considered obese. There are BMI tables in almost every magazine that you read, where you can look up your own BMI.

There is a much easier way, however, to calculate whether you are overweight or not. It is called the **Ideal Weight Formula**:

Females: To calculate your ideal weight, take 100 pounds for your first 5 feet in height. Then you add 5 pounds for each additional inch. For example, if you are 5 feet 2 inches, you should weigh 110 pounds, and that's calculated by taking the 100 pounds for your first 5 feet and 5 pounds for each additional inch, which is another 10 pounds. If you are 15 or more pounds over this ideal weight, then you are considered overweight. If you are 25 or more pounds over this ideal weight, you are considered obese.

Males: Males take 106 pounds for the first 5 feet in height and add 6 pounds for each additional inch. For example, if you are 5 feet 10 inches, then your ideal weight is 166 pounds (5 feet gives you 106 pounds; 10 inches x 6 = 60 more pounds, which gives you a total of 166 pounds). If you are 15 or more pounds over this ideal weight, you are overweight, and if you are 25 or more pounds over your ideal weight, you are obese.

Heart disease and strokes are the leading cause of disability and death in the United States, and being overweight increases your risk of developing either or both of these diseases. People who are overweight are twice as likely to also develop adult-onset diabetes.

By just increasing physical activity to 30 minutes of walking every other day, and losing 5-10% of your current weight, you decrease the risk of heart disease, strokes, and diabetes by more than 50%. Studies have shown that overweight or obese people who exercise regularly and modify their diets have improvements in blood pressure, diabetic control, heart function, blood fats (cholesterol and triglycerides), sleep disorders, and, in general, have improved feelings of well-being and self-esteem. In other words, cutting the total amount of calories and increasing your physical activity is the ideal way to lose and maintain weight and the road toward good health and longevity.

TIP # 65
HIGH ENERGY FOODS

1. Oatmeal

Oatmeal is high in fiber, low in fat, and low in calories. Oatmeal helps to prevent heart disease by lowering your bad cholesterol (LDL) and increasing your good cholesterol (HDL). Many studies have confirmed these findings, and oatmeal is an essential heart-protecting good food. Top your oatmeal off with bananas or berries to increase the flavor and to add extra nutrients and antioxidants to a delicious breakfast snack. Add nonfat milk to your oatmeal for the necessary calcium that your body needs without the added fat present in whole milk or low-fat milk.

2. Yogurt

Calcium-rich yogurt keeps your bones strong and helps to fight off infection by boosting your immune system. The live bacilli in yogurt help to keep your intestinal tract in tip-top shape. All of these benefits are afforded you with either nonfat or low-fat yogurt. You don't need the extra fat content of whole-milk yogurt for it to do its magic. Add fruits to beef up the extra flavor, nutrition, and antioxidant value.

3. Blueberries

Blueberries are chockfull of antioxidants and fiber. They are also low in sugar and calories. Many studies have shown that among all the fruits and vegetables, the antioxidant benefits of blueberries are the greatest. It has also been discovered that blueberry extract has a significant effect on reversing age-related disorders due to its antioxidants. These antioxidents help to neutralize free radical by-products on the conversion of oxygen into energy, which if not neutralized can cause oxidative stress and lead to cell damage. The phytonutrients in blueberries, particularly flavonoids and beta-carotene, seem to have an anti-inflammatory effect, which may even help to prevent the onset of Alzheimer's disease.

4. **Spinach**

Spinach is a great way to increase your fiber, folic acid, vitamin C, and beta-carotene intake. Sautéed with olive oil and a touch of garlic, it makes a great side dish. Spinach can be used in salads or sandwiches instead of boring lettuce. All of the dark leafy greens are heads above the heads of plain lettuce.

Spinach has super healing powers because it is packed with vitamins, antioxidants, and minerals that protect you from many diseases. Spinach contains many antioxidants, including lutein, zeaxanthin, potassium, magnesium, vitamin K, folic acid, and carotenes. Kale is another vegetable which is rich in the antioxidants lutein, and zeaxanthin, which have been reported to protect against age-related cataracts and macular degeneration. Spinach may also lower the risk of strokes, heart disease, osteoporosis, memory loss, and colon cancer. The disease-fighting properties in spinach are better absorbed when spinach is cooked with a little olive oil.

5. **Canned salmon, tuna or sardines**

These three fishes are a great way to increase your essential, heart-healing, inflammation-fighting omega-3 fatty acids. They also provide extra calcium and protein. Add any one to a whole-wheat sandwich with onions, lettuce, tomato, and Dijon mustard, and you have a very tasty lunch snack. Or just add them to a big tossed salad. The ones packed in water are significantly lower in fat; however, if you like the taste of the oil, make sure you drain the can completely of oil and dry the fish off on a paper towel. You will still be getting the yummy taste of the oil and all of the wonderful benefits of the omega-3 fatty acids.

TIP # 66
REALLY GOOD FOODS

1.   **Oranges**
     Oranges (not orange juice) are packed with fiber, vitamin C, folic acid, and other valuable nutrients and antioxidants. Use an orange as a midmorning or midafternoon snack, or just slice them into any salad for a mouthwatering, taste-boosting, delicious treat. Oranges travel well, so put them in your bag or briefcase for an immediate energy boost. Oranges also boost your good cholesterol (HDL) by providing vitamin C, folic acid, and numerous flavinoids to your body. These compounds are thought to prevent cholesterol oxidation, which has been linked to heart disease. Oranges also contain compounds known as liminoids, which seem to alter the characteristics of the lining of the colon, which discourages the growth of cancer in the colon. There has been other research suggesting that oranges may also help to suppress breast, prostate, and lung cancer.

2.   **Whole-grain wheat bread**
     Whole-grain bread is 100% better than white, rye, English muffins, bagels, or just plain wheat bread. Remember, the first ingredient on the label must read "whole-grain wheat flour." Whole-grain bread is packed with fiber, minerals, vitamins, and other essential nutrients. A sandwich with either low-fat turkey, low-fat cheese, or tuna packed in water, plus lettuce, tomato, and cucumber, makes a tasty, crunchy, munchy sandwich.

3.   **Whole-grain cereals**
     Eat high-fiber, whole-grain cereals for breakfast, particularly those with 5 or more grams of fiber per serving. If possible, always choose cereals that state on the ingredient's label: whole grain wheat including the wheat bran or whole grain oats

including the oat bran; or whole grain corn, barley or rice including the bran of that particular cereal grain. You can increase the fiber content of most cereals by adding 1 ½ Tbs. of unprocessed bran or wheat germ, if necessary.

Always add fruits, preferably with the skin, to increase both the fiber content and the nutritional value of cold cereal. Again, make sure that you use nonfat milk, which supplies all of the essential nutrients and calcium without the added fat content present in whole milk or low-fat milk. A daily bowl of cold, whole-grain cereal that supplies 5 or more grams of fiber can cut heart disease risk by up to 35%.

When researchers analyzed the individual effects of three different fiber sources (fruits, vegetables, and cereals), it was found that cereal fiber, more than any other type of fiber, significantly reduced the risk of heart disease. Whole-grain products may increase the body's sensitivity to insulin and thus lower the triglyceride levels. Whole-grain products, especially soy-based cereals, are an important source of phyto-estrogens and may favorably affect blood coagulation activity.

4.   Dried beans, peas, and lentils
Dried beans, peas, and lentils are packed with fiber, folic acid, protein, and antioxidants. This makes them ideal low-calorie, low-fat, high-fiber, high-protein additions to soups or salads. These beans or lentils can be pureed to use as a dip for nonfat chips or tortillas. These foods offer protein and fiber without the cholesterol and fat that is contained in meat. One-half cup of cooked dried beans is about the same as 1 ounce of lean meat. Try substituting beans for meat in your favorite recipe, such as lasagna or chili.

5.   Fruits and vegetables
Eat at least four to five servings of fruits and vegetables each day. Fruits and vegetables are low in fat, and they add flavor and

variety to your diet. They contain fiber, vitamins, minerals, phyto-nutrients, and many beneficial compounds that prevent cardio-vascular disease, stroke, cancer, diabetes, or high cholesterol. The nutrients in fruits and vegetables have been associated with a lower risk of heart disease and a lower risk of stroke.

A study reported in the Journal of the American Medical Associa-tion describes the association between the intake of fruit and veg-etables and ischemic strokes in men and women. This study re-ported that there was an approximately 35% reduction in strokes in men and women who ate between four to five servings of fruit and vegetables daily. The consumption of a variety of vegetables and fruit, for example green leafy vegetables, citrus fruits, crucif-erous vegetables (broccoli and cabbage), and vitamin C-rich fruits and vegetables resulted in the largest decrease in risk.

6.   **Increase omega-3 fats and decrease omega-6 fats**
The American Institute for Cancer Research has recommended that people eat more foods containing omega-3 fats and fewer food containing omega-6 fats. Omega-3 fats are heart healthy fats, which lower blood cholesterol, prevent blood clots, and help to prevent heart attacks. These omega-3 fats also have cancer-inhibiting effects against breast and colon cancer. These healthy omega-3 fats are found in fish oils (sardines, salmon, trout, herring, cod, flounder, sole, haddock) and in walnuts, flaxseed, spinach, broccoli, kale, and canola & olive oils.

Omega-6 fats can be helpful in small amounts by making your blood vessels stronger and help to lower your cholesterol. However, in excess, omega-6 fats are harmful, since they can raise your blood cholesterol, cause dangerous inflammation in your body's cells and prevent the immune system from working properly. They can even speed up the growth of some breast tumors. Avoid cooking oils (corn, soybean, safflower, sunflower and cottonseed oils), salad dressings, and processed foods (cookies, chips, crackers and baked goods).

TIP # 67
REALLY BAD FOODS!

1.   Red meat

Red meat, which is high in fat (cholesterol and saturated fats), is really bad for your arteries. The fat content blocks up the coronary arteries leading to the heart, causing heart disease. It also causes the arteries in the brain to clog up, leading to strokes or TIA's (mini-strokes). The high fat content in meat has also been implicated in the development of cancer of the colon, breast, and prostate gland.

With the added hormones and potential contaminants (for example: mad cow disease), red meat is about the worst food that you can consume. You can get the same protein value without the added fat or detrimental compounds by substituting fish, white meat of chicken, turkey breast, or beans and nuts, and soy-based foods as a substitute for the fat-laden red meat.

2.   Potato chips and French fries

Potato chips are high in saturated fat, trans fats, and salt. These crunchy morsels can provide the body with dangerous levels of omega-6 fatty acids, which can cause your arteries to clog up and can also cause inflammation in the tissues of the body's cells and organs. While you are crunching these crispy delights, say to yourself, "Bad, bad, very bad." Be very afraid!

Fat may not be the only danger lurking in the ever-popular French fries. Besides saturated fats, trans-fats, and tons of calories, a new hidden danger has been discovered in French fries. A recent study has found that frying or baking starchy carbohydrates like potatoes at high temperatures produces a chemical known as *acrylamide*, which is known to cause cancer and reproductive problems in laboratory animals. Many researchers feel that acrylamide poses a real cancer threat in humans. Here's yet another reason to eliminate French fries from your diet. Lose the fat and lower your risk of heart disease, strokes, high blood pressure, and now, even cancer.

3.   Fast foods

Fast foods are really bad foods, especially those sold in fast-food restaurants. One meal consisting of a double cheeseburger, large fries, and large soda is filled with enough calories, fat, sugar, and salt to raise your blood cholesterol and blood pressure and blood sugar to astronomical numbers. Stay away from most fast foods, unless you concentrate on the salad bar with nonfat dressing, or a plain hamburger without sauce or cheese, or grilled chicken without the extra dressings or sauce.

4.   Desserts

Most desserts, including cakes, pies, candies, and ice cream are extremely high in refined sugar. This refined sugar content quickly increases your blood glucose level, which just as quickly increases your pancreas's production of insulin, which in turn stores excess fat in your body's cells. What happens subsequently is a rapid drop in blood sugar and an increase in your hunger level, which causes you to binge-eat on highly refined sugar products. Also, be careful of the so-called diet cakes, pies, cookies, which state they have a low sugar content. These products may have an extremely high fat content and a high number of calories. These highly refined sugar products have essentially no fiber, no nutrients, and no beneficial contents, other than empty calories and should be eliminated from any real diet plan.

Avoid rich bakery foods, such as muffins, doughnuts, sweet rolls, and cakes. Most of these bakery foods contain over 50% fat calories, in addition to the extremely high content of refined sugar. Snacks such as gingersnap cookies, angel food cake, and fruits of all shapes, sizes, and colors will satisfy your sweet tooth without adding excess sugar or fat to your diet. Also, be careful of granola cereals, which may have high sugar content and high levels of fat oils. Instant cooked cereals may also contain high levels of sugar.

5.   Smoked and cured fish and meats and pickled foods

Smoked foods contain many harmful chemicals, such as phenols and nitrates. When cooked and digested, these chemicals form nitrosamines, which are cancer-causing agents. These foods are also high in saturated fats, which can increase your risk for heart disease. Pickled foods also contain nitrates, which are converted to cancer-forming nitrosamines in the digestive tract.

Fruits and vegetables which are rich in vitamin C, A, beta-carotene, and antioxidants, may be able to inhibit the formation of these cancer-causing nitrosamines. So, if you have occasion to eat smoked or cured meats and fish or pickled foods, be sure to add generous amounts of veggies and fruits to your meal to counteract the harmful effects of these bad chemicals.

6.   Salt

The National Academy of Sciences now recommends that you limit your salt or sodium intake to no more than 2,000 mg per day. Although some salt is essential in the diet for maintaining the fluid balance of the body, excess salt intake can cause a permanent elevation of blood pressure by interfering with the kidneys' ability to eliminate salt from the body. This excess accumulation of sodium causes the body to retain more liquid and subsequently increases the volume of blood. This, in turn, makes the heart work harder, causing a rise in blood pressure. In susceptible people, this may result in permanent hypertension and premature death from strokes or heart attacks.

7.   Alcohol

Excess alcohol can cause liver disease, brain damage, nerve disorders, strokes, heart disease, hypertension, damage to the reproductive organs, enlargement of the spleen, hemorrhages of the esophagus, and liver and pancreatic cancer. While a small glass of red wine daily has been shown to be heart-protective, excess alcohol can lead to many diseases and premature death. And don't forget, alcohol contains 7 calories for each gram of alcohol. So excessive alcohol intake is both detrimental to your health and your waistline.

8.   Caffeine

Excess caffeine consumption causes marked fatigue after the initial stimulating effect of the caffeine wears off. Caffeine also has an adverse effect on the cardiovascular and nervous systems. It can cause a rapid heartbeat, palpitations, elevation of blood pressure, and an irritation of all of the body's nerve endings. This can result in headaches, nervousness, sweats, tremors, mental confusion, anxiety, and even paranoid behavior. Following these adverse effects is marked lethargy, which saps the body of its vital energy. One or two cups of coffee or tea daily probably will not cause any of these nasty side effects, provided you do not have an exaggerated reaction to caffeine. Remember also, that excess caffeine intake has an appetite-stimulating effect.

9.   Smoking - O.K., So it's not a food!

Even though smoking is not considered a food, many addicted people substitute it for food. Smoking causes fatigue by impairing the delivery of oxygen to the cells of all of your body's organs. Smoking increases the level of carbon monoxide in your blood, which damages the heart and lungs, leading to cardiovascular disease, pulmonary disorders, and cancer. Smoking destroys vitamin C in the body, which impairs the immune system and decreases your energy level. Also, smoking causes premature wrinkling of the skin and a sallow-appearing complexion. I always tell my patients who are attempting to stop smoking and are concerned about gaining weight, "You can always lose the additional weight that you gain after you stop smoking. However, you can never undo the harmful effects of cigarettes."

TIP # 68
SECRET WEIGHT-LOSS TIPS
FOR SENIORS!

WHY SENIORS GAIN WEIGHT EASILY

· Seniors gain weight easier as they get older because of a slow-down in the body's basal metabolism.

· It therefore takes longer for a senior to digest food than it does for a younger person.

· As we age, we develop a slight deficiency of certain digestive enzymes, which makes it more difficult to digest food, particularly fat.

· Fat in a senior's diet therefore causes her or him to gain weight more easily because of this inability to digest and metabolize fat quickly.

· So fat in a senior's diet is just about the worst thing that he or she can do to lose weight and stay healthy.

· The very worst types of diets for seniors are the low carbohydrate, high fat diets. They don't work and they are very unhealthy, particularly in the elderly.

SECRET FORMULA PART #1:
30 GRAMS OF FAT

· Fat contains 9 calories per gram whereas both carbohydrate and protein contain only 4 calories per gram.

· Excess fat in the diet causes heart disease, diabetes, vascular disease and breast and uterine cancer.

· Less fat in the diet results in more storage fat being burned as fuel, so both you and your fat cells become thinner.

· 1 pound of body fat contains 3,500 calories, which makes it very easy to gain weight when you eat fat, since fat contains more than twice the number of calories as carbohydrate and protein.

· Fat is the number 1 killer of both your heart and your figure.

· Eat no more than 30 grams of total fat calories daily to lose weight.

· Consult a chart for the total grams of fat in various foods and keep a record of what you eat.

· To maintain your ideal weight, eat no more than 35 grams of total fat calories daily.

SECRET FORMULA PART #2:
30 GRAMS OF FIBER

· Fiber helps you to lose weight because of the slower emptying of the stomach and makes you feel full earlier.

· Fiber foods contain fewer calories for their large volume so that it fills you up without filling you out.

· Fiber has a high bulk ratio, which makes your hunger center satisfied more quickly.

· Fiber has the ability to absorb lots of water and therefore regulates the progression of food through the digestive system.

· Fiber can also block fat absorption and help to burn fat and calories eaten.

· Fiber helps to lower blood cholesterol and also decreases the risk of heart disease, hypertension and stroke.

· Fiber helps to keep the digestive system healthy.

· Fruits, vegetables and whole grains are not only high in fiber but also contain many nutrients and antioxidants.

· To lose weight, eat at least 30 grams of fiber daily.

· Consult a chart for total grams of fiber in various foods and keep a record of what you eat.

· To maintain your ideal weight eat no less than 25 grams of fiber daily.

SECRET FORMULA PART # 3:
30 MINUTES WALKING DAILY

- Walking is the ideal aerobic exercise for good health, fitness and weight-loss without the dangers of strenuous exercise.
- Walking burns approximately 3,500 calories per hour, so you can lose 1 pound of body fat for every 10 hours you walk.
- Strenuous exercise burns primarily carbohydrates to produce energy and does very little to help you lose weight.
- As strenuous exercise burns carbohydrates it produces a drop in blood sugar, which actually increases your appetite.
- Slow, continuous, moderate activity like walking burns primarily fat stored in the body and is the best exercise for sustained weight-loss. You lose more fat and less muscle.
- Walking increases the body's metabolic rate, which helps to burn calories at a faster rate.
- Walking as an aerobic exercise re-directs blood away from the stomach to the exercising muscles and decreases appetite.
- Walking regulates the brain's appetite center. Walking before a meal decreases the appetite.
- Walking has the added benefit of decreasing the risk of heart disease, hypertension, stroke and certain forms of cancer.
- A 30-minute brisk walk daily will burn enough calories to help you lose weight easily. 15-minutes twice a day is just as good.
- Once you've reached your ideal weight, take a day off each week and rest.

TIP # 69
STAY AWAY FROM THE SCALE

Remember, no one loses weight in a straight line. When you are on a diet, you initially lose weight, and then your weight loss levels off. This occurs even though you are eating exactly the same amount as you were when you lost the initial weight. This leveling-off period or *plateau* is the single most hazardous part of any diet program. The reason is that once this plateau is reached, you begin to become discouraged, and you'll say, "I'm still on the same diet, but I haven't lost a pound in over a week." Discouragement leads to frustration, and next you'll say, "The heck with the diet. I may as well enjoy myself and eat something I really like, since I haven't lost weight anyway." At this point, 90 percent of all diets are doomed to failure, since the weight-loss pattern now reverses itself and becomes a *weight gain pattern.*

If you can stick out this plateau period, which incidentally is *always temporary*, you'll be surprised to see that the weight-loss begins to pick up speed again. It may take a week or two, at the most, but if you are patient, you will again start to lose those unwanted pounds. No one has ever satisfactorily explained this plateau period; however, physiologists believe that it is probably due to *a temporary readjustment of the body's metabolism* in response to the initial weight-loss. No matter what the reason is, however, you will always break through the plateau period, providing you don't become discouraged or frustrated. Weight-loss will again resume its downward progress toward your ideal weight goal.

This plateau period is one of the main reasons that I insist that my patients do not weigh themselves daily. In fact, *weighing yourself every day is hazardous to your diet.* The reason for this is twofold. *First,* when you weigh yourself daily and see that you are losing weight, you become happy and elated, and subconsciously you will eat to celebrate. *Secondly,* if you see that you are not losing weight as fast as you "think you should," you become depressed and anxious, and sometime during that day you will subconsciously eat because of frustration. So, the rule of thumb is: *The more you weigh yourself, the more you eat!*

Believe me, it is true. I've seen my patients go through this frustrating daily weighing process thousands of times. No one dieting should weigh oneself more than once a week, and then you will get a true measure of the effectiveness of your diet. If you must weigh yourself, then Wednesday is the best day to weigh yourself each week. Monday and Friday are the worst days for weighing in, since they follow and precede the weekend and lead to frustrating eating binges. It took a long time to gain all that weight; you can't take it off overnight. Be patient!

TIP # 70
POPCORN: HIGH FIBER, LOW FAT, LOW CALORIE SNACK

Without the added salt, oil, and butter, popcorn is probably one of the best diet snacks available. It is *low in calories and cholesterol, and high in fiber*. It consequently fills you up without adding extra calories and provides 2 grams of fiber per 1-½ cups. One cup of popcorn contains only 25 calories. The *electric hot-air popper* is, by far, the most efficient way to prepare popcorn. Since it uses no oil, there are no added fats, and there is no cleanup necessary. These hot-air poppers can produce great quantities of popcorn in a relatively short period of time. This electric appliance is a must for your low-cholesterol, high-fiber, low calorie diet. Most microwaveable popcorns contain considerable fat; however, several newer products are available in low-fat varieties. Always check the label.

There are a number of combinations that can be used with popcorn to add flavor and variety to this low-calorie snack:

1. Popcorn can be eaten as a breakfast cereal with fruit, skim milk, and a teaspoon of wheat germ.
2. Popcorn croutons: Popcorn can be used in salads and soups in place of croutons.
3. Popcorn and peanuts: Popcorn and peanuts (unsalted, dry-roasted peanuts) can be an excellent evening snack with a glass of diet soda.
4. Popcorn, peanuts, and raisins: Same as above.
5. Apple and popcorn: Slices of apple mixed with popcorn can be an ideal snack.
6. Cooking with popcorn: Apple popcorn crisp, chili popcorn, parmesan popcorn, garlic popcorn, peanut butter popcorn balls, raisin or cinnamon popcorn, fruit and popcorn balls are examples of serving ideas.

TIP # 71
DIET TIPS FOR SLIM HIPS

1.   Don't skip meals.

Skipping meals lowers your blood sugar, which brings on cravings for high-carbohydrate, high-calorie foods. In many people, going hungry can bring on "hunger headaches" similar to migraine-type headaches. Eating three to four, or even five small meals per day is far superior to eating one or two large meals. If your blood sugar remains constant, then you're less likely to overeat and gain weight.

Have you ever noticed thin, wiry people who seem to be eating all the time, but never get fat? That's because they eat small, frequent meals, which are lower in calories and their metabolism seems to burn them up at a faster rate, rather than having to deal with a large number of calories all at once. And besides, small, frequent meals are usually consumed by active, rather than sedentary, people. The high-calorie, large meal eater usually eats and sits and sits and eats. And when they are finished eating, they are too bloated to get up and move around. The small meat eater is up and about before you know it.

2.   Eliminate the fat in your diet.

Most people do not realize the amount of fat calories that they consume each day. The first order of business is to find the fat in your diet and eliminate it. Everyone knows that there's fat in bacon, lunchmeats, eggs, butter, ice cream, milk, and cheese. But not everyone realizes that there's considerable fat in donuts, cakes, pies, muffins, margarine, mayonnaise, chicken and tuna salad, coffee creamers, yogurt, cream cheese, and cottage cheese – (even the ones marked low-fat).

Your body metabolizes fats and carbohydrates together in a set ratio governed genetically by your individual body's metabolism. When you restrict the number of fat calories that you consume, then your body's metabolism automatically controls the amount of refined carbohydrate calories that you actually eat. By restricting the fat calories eaten, you crave less refined carbohydrates in your diet. The combination of less fat eaten, combined with less refined carbohydrates craved, makes it next to impossible for you to put on excess weight. So, when you *eat less fat you're less likely to get fat.* Sounds simple? It is!

3.   Avoid eating fast and fast-food eating.

If you're a fast eater or a fast-food eater – watch out! When you consume food at a rapid pace, you have a greater tendency to consume excess calories by overeating. The reason for this is that it takes 15-20 minutes for the brain's appetite regulator (the appestat) to receive the signals that your body's stomach is full. If you eat your meal rapidly in 5 or 10 minutes, as you often do in fast-food restaurants, then your appestat will never know that you've eaten.

Subsequently, you'll still be as hungry as you were before you wolfed down that bacon double-cheeseburger. And you'll probably order a milkshake and a large order of French fries. By the time you get those down the hatch, your brain will just be receiving the first signals that you're full from the original double bacon cheeseburger that you ate in the first five minutes. Well, it's too late by then. The appestat will never know that you've eaten 620 calories and 38 grams of fat (bacon double cheeseburger), and 590 calories and 30 grams of fat (large french fries), and 400 calories and 9 grams of fat (milkshake). Only your waistline, hips, and thighs will be the wiser.

4.   Chew food thoroughly and eat foods that need chewing.

Foods that require a good bit of chewing, like apples, corn, celery, carrots, salads, cucumber, raw vegetables (cauliflower, broccoli, string beans, radishes, etc.), are excellent diet foods, since they take time to chew, and consequently the brain's appetite regulating mechanism (appestat) is satisfied long before you've had a chance to consume too many calories.

An apple a day not only keeps the doctor away, but it also keeps the fat away from your body. Apples are high-fiber foods, which not only take longer to eat than most other comparably sized foods, but have many nutritional advantages over low-fiber foods. One reason the appestat is appeased early is the time that it takes for you to eat an apple. The other reason is that the high fiber content of apples and similar high-fiber foods produces more bulk in the stomach, making you feel full faster.

5.   Don't skip breakfast.

People who never eat breakfast usually make up for it sometime during the day, and then some. By the time lunch comes, your low blood sugar gives you a ravenous appetite and you're sure to overeat. Or, you may get hungry long before lunchtime arrives, and you'll end up stuffing donuts and coffee into your face. Remember, too, that caffeine is an appetite stimulant, and you should be careful not to drink too much coffee or tea. People who skip breakfast seem to make up for it threefold by snacking midmorning, midafternoon, and late evening. This appears to be due to the fact that the metabolism seems to slow down later in the day in non-breakfast eaters.

The body reacts to a lack of breakfast because it thinks you are starving, and so it slows down your metabolism in an attempt to conserve calories. This results in sluggishness and fatigue, which, in turn, cause you to "just eat something" in order to feel better. Eating speeds up the metabolism and elevates the blood sugar, and lo and behold, you feel better. Then the blood sugar rapidly drops again, and you feel fatigued again, and so you eat again. This is called *functional hypoglycemia* or low blood sugar, which results from just skipping meals. Other causes of hypoglycemia are the result of excess alcohol, caffeine, nicotine, sugar, and stress.

6.   Dieting can be fun!

The most important part of any successful diet is starting it. Once you've made up your mind to begin your diet, you're halfway there. You must also be able to have fun with your diet. A low fat, high fiber, moderate protein diet does not require much discipline, since it's easy to follow and you see results quickly. In fact, the diet is fun to follow, since you know you are losing weight by eating healthful, colorful, exciting, good-tasting foods. Try some; it's fun!

TIP # 72
FIGURE FOODS

Foods that are good for you are also good for your figure. Most of the foods that promote good health are also foods that help you stay slim and trim.

Fruits – are high in fiber and low in calories. They fill you up without filling you out. Fruits satisfy the appestat by taking longer to consume, and they promote good bowel health by providing adequate fiber, which in turn also reduces your appetite. Fruits are not only low-fat, low-calorie foods, but they are especially rich in *potassium*. Potassium is an essential element, which appears to have blood pressure lowering properties. In a recent medical study, potassium-rich foods reduced the risk of strokes by more than 30% in individuals who had known hypertension.

Fruits are also good sources of pectin, a fiber found in many fruits and vegetables. This particular type of fiber helps to lower blood cholesterol. Many of these fruits, which are high in pectin, also contain vitamin C, which helps the pectin lower cholesterol even more than pectin alone. Vitamin C also is important in boosting our immune system, and also has cancer-inhibiting factors built into its structure.

Fish – Studies show that diets rich in fish lower blood pressure 15-20% in hypertensive men. A study conducted at the Cardiovascular Research Institute in West Germany showed that men with mild hypertension who ate three cans of mackerel per week had a significant reduction in their blood pressures. Other studies in the United States have confirmed these findings.

Fish oil has been shown to reduce blood fats and, consequently, slow the formation of deposits of cholesterol in the arteries. In a study at the University of Chicago, monkeys on a diet high in fish oil developed less cholesterol deposits in their arteries than monkeys fed a diet high in saturated fat and coconut oil. The monkeys fed fish oil also had lower total cholesterol and LDL cholesterol levels than the monkeys fed the high saturated fat diet. Another study conducted at Harvard Medical School appears to indicate that fish oils also have a cancer-inhibiting factor. In a study of rats with breast cancer, fish oils seem to slow the spread of the disease significantly more than diets high in saturated fat or polyunsaturated fats, and even more than just a low-fat diet.

It appears that the omega-3 fatty acids present in fish oils are the ingredient responsible for the cholesterol-lowering and cancer-inhibiting effects. Fish is not only low in saturated fats and calories, but it's high in omega-3 fatty acids that help to lower both your cholesterol and triglyceride levels. Eat fish two to three times per week for a healthy heart and a slim body. Many recent studies at major universities have also found that the omega-3 oils help to prevent platelet cells in the blood from getting sticky, decreasing the tendency for blood clots to form. Eskimos and the Japanese, who consume lots of fish, don't typically have heart attacks from fat-clogged arteries.

Omega-3 fatty acids found in fish oil also have been found to be essential for brain function. Recent studies have found that a lack of omega-3 fatty acids may be responsible for learning disabilities, memory loss, difficulty concentrating, and certain degenerative diseases, including Alzheimer's disease. In a recent study, age-related memory decline was halted or slowed down considerably in women who ate ¾ ounce of fish every other day. New evidence has also shown that fish oils may even help in the treatment of major depression and other neurologic and psychiatric disorders.

Cereal grain, especially oats and bran – provide water-soluble fiber that helps to lower both cholesterol and triglyceride levels. These high-fiber cereals also promote good bowel health by reducing constipation and preventing hemorrhoids, diverticulitis, appendicitis, and varicose veins, and reducing the incidence of colon cancer.

Fowl – Lean white meat of turkey and chicken is low in calories and fat, and high in protein, promoting good health and a slim figure. Make sure you remove the skin, which contains high amounts of saturated fat, before eating fowl.

Onions, garlic, and peppers – help to lower levels of blood fats, lower blood pressure, and help to make the blood less likely to clot. These foods contain certain natural chemical substances that actually thin your blood and help to reduce your appetite.

Vegetables – It's important to eat more vegetables of the cabbage family, particularly broccoli, cauliflower, spinach, Brussels sprouts, and squash. These foods are not only high in fiber, but they are also high in both vitamin A and C, and are rich in phytonutrients, which are cancer-fighting agents. Many vegetables rich in potassium are sweet potatoes, squash, spinach, beets, tomatoes, and green peppers. Boiling destroys more than 35-40% of the potassium in vegetables, so remember to eat more raw vegetables and steam or microwave vegetables, rather than boil them, in order to reduce potassium loss. Vegetables are low in calories and contain no fat and are great foods for weight loss and weight maintenance.

Carrots and leafy green vegetables contain beta-carotene and other carotenes, which are chemical precursors to vitamin A. Beta-carotene is converted to vitamin A in the body. Vitamin A inhibits compounds called free radicals in the body, which may cause normal cells to turn cancerous. Vitamin A also maintains the integrity of the lungs and the intestinal tract. Beta-carotene appears to have a protective effect against both lung and colon cancer. A recent study conducted at the New York State University in Buffalo found that people with lung cancer had significantly lower blood levels of beta-carotene than a similar number of people who were free of the disease. Similar studies have shown that patients with colon cancer also have lower levels of beta-carotene than a comparable number of healthy individuals.

VIII.
CALORIE-
BLASTING
TIPS

TIP # 73
CALCIUM BURNS FAT & BUILDS BONES

Several new studies have shown that people who drink two glasses of skim milk or eat two cups of yogurt or one serving of cheese per day, can lose an average of 1-½ pounds per month, with no additional change in their diets. It is believed that the mineral calcium present in these foods burns stored fat, while promoting the buildup of more muscle tissue. Also, it is thought that the protein content in milk, yogurt and cheese replaces the fat stored in the fat cells by a unique process of providing extra protein to the body's cells. This combination of calcium and protein which is present in milk, yogurt and cheese helps the body to burn fat and store protein.

Another new study suggests that the calcium found in these foods actually blocks fat storage in the cells that plump up your abdomen, thighs and hips. This calcium also has the added advantage of increasing your good HDL cholesterol and decreasing your bad LDL cholesterol. Non-fat milk and low-fat cheeses and non-fat or low-fat yogurts have the same amount of minerals, vitamins, protein and calcium as whole milk without the added fat content. And, as far as your diet is concerned, fat-free milk contains only 80 calories per glass and is packed with 220 mg. of calcium.

Calcium is important in the formation and maintenance of healthy bones. More than 60% of people do not consume the recommended daily intake of calcium. If you are between 20 and 45 years of age, you need at least 500 to 750 mg of calcium daily, and if you're over 45, you need 1,000 to 1,200 mg per day, whether you are a man or a woman.

To accomplish the necessary calcium requirement in the diet, eat at least two servings of nonfat dairy products daily (milk, yogurt, cheese). Also try calcium-fortified orange juice, cereals, and soy milk for added calcium in the diet. Canned salmon and sardines, with their bones left in, add a high level of calcium to your diet.

It is also essential that you get enough vitamin D in your diet for the proper absorption of calcium. Skim or 1% milk is fortified with the same amount of vitamin D as contained in whole milk, which helps the calcium contained in the milk to be absorbed properly. Sunlight also provides vitamin D, which is absorbed through your skin. You need at least 20 minutes of sunlight daily to get enough vitamin D in your body to absorb calcium properly. In winter, however, when sunlight is at a premium, it is necessary to take a vitamin D supplement.

If you take a calcium supplement, be sure that it contains vitamin D in the formula. If you need 1,000 mg per day, take the supplements in smaller, divided doses for better absorption. Those supplements made of calcium citrate are absorbed more completely than other forms of calcium, such as calcium carbonate.

Vitamins C and K are also important in keeping your bones healthy. Foods rich in vitamin C include tomatoes, peppers, blueberries, strawberries, oranges, lemons, limes, and other fruits. Foods rich in vitamin K include dark green, leafy vegetables like broccoli, asparagus, spinach, collard greens, and bok choy.

Low carbohydrate diets that are essentially high in fat and protein can tend to leach calcium out of your bones. Carbonated beverages also cause your bones to leak calcium because the phosphorus content of these drinks needs calcium to be neutralized in the bloodstream. Alcohol, as well, in excess can cause thinning of the bones. Extremely low calorie diets that eliminate dairy products can also lead to thinning of the bones.

Walking and mild weightbearing exercises are essential to keeping bones healthy. By combining walking and weightbearing exercises with a high calcium diet (from nonfat dairy products), you will be able to lose weight easily, shape up your muscles, firm up your figure, and help keep your bones strong and healthy. Low-fat or nonfat dairy products help to cut your appetite by satisfying the brain's appetite control mechanism (appestat) without consuming large amounts of calories. Also, the protein content of these non-fat or low-fat dairy products also keep your appetite level satisfied for longer periods of time. Both the calcium content and the protein content of these foods are important factors in a healthy, effective weight-loss program.

TIP # 74
JUNK FOODS – THE BEST OF
THE WORST!

Unfortunately, there are lots of times when you're placed in a position where you just can't eat healthy. For instance, you are really hungry and you're waiting at the airport for a flight, or you're already on your flight and the selection of foods is pretty grim. Maybe you are at a sports event or at a movie, and your choices of foods are really limited. How about at someone's party or during a boring meeting at work? The situations are endless where you are hungry and the choices for good nutritious, low-calorie foods are just not available. What you have to do, short of starving, is to make the best choices from the worst foods available. Let's look at some examples of the best of the worst foods.

Tip: **You have to choose between pretzels, chips, or mixed nuts**.

Pretzels are low in fat and calories; however, they're also low in protein and fiber, so even though they're a good initial snack, you're bound to be hungry sooner.

Chips are high in fat and calories and low in fiber and protein, so they are a lose-lose combination. Whether they're potato chips or corn chips or nachos, they usually have tons of fat and little nutritious value.

Peanuts, on the other hand, are higher in fat and calories than pretzels; however, they have enough protein and fiber to keep your hunger at bay until you can get a really healthy meal. They're **"the best of the worst"** choices.

Tip: **What about if your only choice is between a hot dog, a hamburger, or a slice of pizza?**

Both the **hot dog and the hamburger** are filled with lots of saturated fat; however, their only saving feature is their high protein content. However, who really knows what unknown animal parts are in a hot dog, and who really knows what additives or contaminants are contained in that juicy hamburger?

Pizza, on the other hand, is high in fat and calories; however, it does contain protein and calcium from the cheese and fiber and antioxidants, particularly lycopene, found in the tomato sauce. Here, clearly, is **"the best of the worst"** choices. Make sure that you don't add pepperoni to your slice. Otherwise, this best becomes another worst.

Tip: **How about the choice between a muffin, a doughnut, or a bagel with cream cheese?**

Both the **doughnut and muffin** are loaded with fat and calories, with little or no fiber or protein, unless it is a bran muffin, which is still high in fat and calories.

The **bagel** with cream cheese comes out the clear winner of "the best of the worst" choices in this particular case. Try to scrape off as much of the cream cheese as possible, and if possible scoop out the bagel. In any event, the cream cheese does provide calcium and protein, and there is some fiber in the bagel, especially if you can get a whole-wheat bagel, which in most settings is impossible. Still, there's no doubt this is still **"the best of the worst"** of the choices available.

Tip: **What about choosing between a chocolate candy bar, peanut butter and cheese crackers, or a bag of popcorn?**

The **candy bar** is usually loaded with lots of fat, most of which is saturated fat. It also usually contains between 250-300 calories and approximately 10-15 grams of total fat. Clearly, this is the big loser from this threesome.

The **peanut butter and cheese crackers** are high in refined carbs, fat, and calories, although not as high as the candy bar. Its only redeeming quality is its 3-4 grams of protein. Not great, but a better choice than the candy bar.

"**The best of the worst**" in this category is clearly the bag of **popcorn**. The popcorn does have fiber (approximately 2 grams per small bag) and is considerably lower in calories than the candy bar or peanut butter and cheese crackers. It still has plenty of carbs, but it satisfies your appetite longer because of the fiber and air bulk of the popcorn. If you add butter, then "the best of the worst" choice becomes the worst of the worst.

Tip: **Now, we come to the two favorites served at most parties, cake or ice cream.**

Cake is clearly the big loser here because it is packed with calories, fat, and refined sugars. There is clearly no redeeming quality to cake, particularly birthday cake with all of that rich, gooey icing.

Ice cream is definitely "the best of the worst" of these two choices, since it does contain calcium, potassium, and protein. Most of the time, there won't be a choice of low-fat ice cream at a party, so just a small scoop of ice cream is your "**best of the worst**" choice because it is loaded with fat, particularly saturated fat.

If, by chance, there is a choice of **fruit** at a party, then this would jump to the front of the list as "the best" choice. Low in calories, high in fiber and nutrition, fruit always comes out the clear winner.

TIP # 75
WEIGHT-LOSS MYTHS

Myth No. 1 – **The more you perspire, the more calories you burn, and the more weight you lose.**

This is a myth because some people just perspire more than others do. Extra sweating doesn't mean that you're burning extra calories. The key to burning more calories and losing more weight is twofold. One, it's the intensity of your workout that determines how many calories you burn. If you're breathing hard and your muscles feel sore, then you're burning extra calories. Secondly, and actually more importantly, is the duration of your exercise. Moderate, low-intensity exercises, like walking for 30 to 45 minutes, burn more calories than short-term strenuous exercises, without the muscle aches or the heavy breathing. By increasing the basal metabolic rate for a longer period of time, the body burns calories at a steady rate while exercising, and even continues to burn calories, at a lower rate, after the exercise is finished. This is because the basal metabolic rate doesn't slow down immediately after your longer duration moderate exercise. Moderate, steady exercise, like walking, again wins the fitness race.

Myth No. 2 – **Lifting heavy weight either on machines or free weights, burns more calories than lifting light to moderate weights.**

Lifting heavy weight does burn more calories initially; however, since this activity cannot be continued for a long time, calories are only burned short-term. Besides, heavy weight lifting is essentially unhealthy, since it can cause muscle and ligament tears and various other tendon injuries. Interestingly enough, studies have shown that lifting heavy weights may contribute to the development of high blood pressure, since this is an anaerobic exercise, which does not produce oxygenation of all of the body's cells, like aerobic exercises do.

Strength-training exercises, using light to moderate weights, on the other hand, can be continued for a longer duration, which leads to the steady burning of calories. It actually boosts your overall metabolism. This, in turn, leads to weight- loss and the gradual sculpting of muscles for a better, not bigger, figure. Also, these strength-training exercises help to prevent thinning of the bones as we age (osteoporosis). These exercises build more muscle, which burns more calories than fat, even after you stop exercising. Again, we have an example of slow and steady wins the fitness and weight-reducing race. And in this particular case, the muscle and figure-improving race.

***Myth No. 3* – A morning workout like running burns more calories than at any other time of day, and subsequently you will lose more weight quickly.**

Calories burned are dependent on the type and duration of exercise that you do. It has nothing to do with the time of day. Your body can't differentiate between a morning or an evening workout. All that your body knows is how many calories you've burned by the duration and the type of exercise you are doing at any particular time of day. The same formula holds, no matter when you exercise. It takes burning 3,500 calories to lose one pound of body fat. This can take a day, or a week, or a month; the calories that are burned are cumulative. In other words, if you burn 350 calories a day walking, you will lose a pound of body fat in ten days (350 calories x 10 days = 3,500 calories burned).

***Myth No. 4* – Anything that you eat in the evening will turn to fat, since you're inactive in the evening and while you're sleeping.**

This is another myth regarding weight-loss. It doesn't make any difference when you eat. It's the total number of calories that you consume daily vs. the total number of calories that you burn daily that determines weight-loss or weight gain. Your body does not differentiate calories eaten during the day or in the evening, only how many calories you have eaten on that particular day. The only disadvantage to eating late in the evening is if you have a condition known as acid reflux, and in that particular case, this could precipitate heartburn. If you do have reflux, it is certainly essential to have this checked by your physician.

Myth No. 5 – **Running and strenuous aerobic exercises are the best way to lose weight.**

Strenuous exercises burn primarily carbohydrates during the first two-thirds of your workout, and then begin to burn fat only during the last one-third of the workout. Walking and moderate exercises, on the other hand, burn fat during the first two-thirds of your workout, and then burn carbohydrates in the last third of the workout. You can clearly see that you will burn more calories (fat has 9 calories per gram compared with carbohydrate, which has 4 calories per gram) by moderate exercises like walking.

Strenuous exercises are not only ineffective in a weight-reduction program, but they are dangerous, since they contribute to muscle and ligament injuries, strains and sprains, and have even been known to cause more serious problems like heart attacks and strokes.

A recent study from the University of Pittsburgh found that women who rated their exercise as moderate lost a comparable amount of weight, if not more weight, than those women who exercised vigorously. It's the total duration of activity, and not the intensity of activity, that burns more calories. Weight-loss occurs more gradually and more effectively in a moderate exercise program like walking. Walking also contributes to the maintenance of weight-loss for as long as you continue your walking program.

Myth No. 6 – **Fasting for one or two days can help you to lose weight.**

On the contrary, fasting does not lead to weight-loss, because your body metabolism slows down considerably. The body is attempting to conserve calories, since it thinks that you are starving to death, and wants to prevent you from getting sick. So, calories are burned at a much slower rate and it's unlikely you will lose any weight at all by fasting. Besides, once you resume your food intake, your body's metabolism remains in its slow-down phase until it's sure that you're not starving. During this time, most of the calories you eat get stored in fat cells and you are likely to gain extra weight instead of losing weight.

Myth No. 7 – Vegetarian diets are healthier and help you lose weight more easily than non-vegetarian diets.

Again, it's the total number of calories consumed daily that determines weight-loss or weight gain. This occurs regardless of whether you are eating vegetables or meat. The only problem with a strict vegetarian diet that doesn't allow meat, fish, fowl, or dairy is that you are losing essential vitamins and minerals that your body needs. You must supplement these losses with a multivitamin and mineral supplement. Also, strict vegetarians can become protein-deficient and have to rely on nuts, legumes, and soy for their protein. Strict vegetarians also tend to consume many refined carbohydrate, processed foods, which are high in fat and calories. So, it's unlikely that a strict vegetarian diet is better for weight-loss than a more balanced, low-calorie, low-fat, moderate protein and complex carbohydrate-type of diet.

TIP # 76
HOW ABOUT A SALAD SANDWICH?

How would you like an egg, tuna or chicken salad sandwich for lunch with a twist? The twist is that there's absolutely no bread whatsoever in this sandwich. Salads are great diet lunches but you have to eat them with a fork. It's obviously more fun to bite into a great tasting chewy sandwich. Well, here's a salad sandwich for you. Take a large piece of Ice-Burg lettuce or Romaine and use it like a pita wrap. Fill it up with your favorite salad ingredients, roll up the lettuce or Romaine and pin it with a tooth-pick until you're ready to eat it. You get the great crunch-factor of eating a sandwich without the bread.

Egg salad is great for a lettuce wrap. Use two or three fresh hard-boiled eggs and discard the yolk from one of them. This lowers the cholesterol count without reducing the taste of the egg salad. Chop in some fresh dill and celery to boost the taste of the egg salad. Be sure to use non-fat or very low fat mayo when preparing your egg salad. Add sliced tomato or cucumber to improve the texture, taste and crunch factor of your salad sandwich.

Tip: Egg yolk is not as bad as it was once thought to be. Egg yolk contains two chemicals called lutein and xanthine, which are important in shielding the retina of the eye from the harmful effects of ultraviolet light from the sun. These two chemicals also appear to reduce both the risk of developing cataracts and macular degeneration of the eye. Since eggs are low in total saturated fat, there appears to be no direct link between the cholesterol content of egg yolk and heart disease. Eggs are also low in calories and are chocked full of nutrition, including protein, vitamins A, B12, folic acid and riboflavin. For good nutrition and weight-loss, eat an egg every other day and on alternate days eat two egg whites from hard-boiled eggs or make an egg white omelet with fresh veggies.

Tuna, chicken or crab meat salads also make tasty, nutritious low calorie, high protein lettuce wraps. When these wraps are made with non- or very low fat mayo, they are great tasting, crunchy salad sandwiches. Add celery, cucumber and tomato to boost the taste and flavor of your lettuce wrap.

Chicken salad can also be spiced up with a little Indian curry powder, lemongrass and lime. Also, a tasty addition to chicken salad is to add grapes, pecans or walnuts and apples.

Crab salad can also be made with lemon juice, watercress, Dijon mustard and a touch of olive oil.

Tip: Salad sandwiches are low in calories and high in nutrition. Here's one instance when even a second helping won't interfere with your weight-loss program. This is just one more of the 100 Best Weight- Loss Tips.

MORE SALAD CHOICES WITHOUT THE WRAPS

Here are some healthy, nutritious salad ingredients that are low in calories and fat, and contain good sources of protein and are packed with vitamins, minerals, and phytonutrients. You can mix and match any of these ingredients, or any other similar salad ingredients, for your really good salad.

- One cup of Boston lettuce or one cup baby spinach (30 calories, high in vitamin K and folate).

- 3 Tbs. (1/4 cup) raisins (70 calories, 2 grams of fiber, 310 mg of potassium, 0 grams of fat).

- 1 Tbs. roasted sunflower or sesame seeds or walnuts (40 calories, 3 grams of good fat, 1 gram of fiber, vitamin E 100 I.U).

- One-third cup tofu cubes (30 calories, 1 gram of fat, 10 mg of iron).

- One-third cup sliced carrots (10 calories, 0 grams of fat, high in vitamin A, B, and carotene).

- One-third cup broccoli (10 calories, 0 grams of fat, high in vitamin K).

- 1 Tbs. feta cheese (25 calories, 2 gram of fat, 50 mg calcium).

- One-third cup sliced beets (10 calories, 0 grams of fat, 1 gram fiber).

- One-third cup chickpeas (48 calories, 0.5 grams fat, 1 gram fiber, good source of vitamin B_6 and B_{12}).

- One-third cup alfalfa sprouts (3 calories, 0 grams of fat, 0.5 grams fiber).

- One sliced egg, white only (20 calories, 0 grams of fat, good source of protein and vitamin D).

- Three medium black olives (21 calories, 4 grams of good olive oil fat, 1 gram fiber).

- Add one sliced chicken breast or a small can of tuna packed in water to the salad to make it an entire meal, which is packed with lean protein.

TIP # 77
PEER PRESSURE TO EAT MORE

Recently, research shows that you eat more when you are dining with more people. This is especially true if the people you are eating with consume larger amounts of food. Your appetite goes into overdrive when you are with several people, especially if you are talking and enjoying yourself with friends. What happens is that with the excitement of dining with friends, your appetite mechanism doesn't shut off easily, since you're talking and having fun. Before you know it, you're eating much more than you should have eaten, while not realizing the total amount of food that you have consumed.

Plan in advance if you're going to have dinner with friends. Order a low-fat, low-calorie meal, regardless of what your dinner companions order. Concentrate on taking small bites and eating slowly while eating with friends. Also, stop your meal while talking, so that you're not consuming mass quantities of food without realizing this fact. If you're a woman dining with a man, you should know that men can eat much more food than you can without gaining weight. Who said life was fair! Men burn more calories quickly because of testosterone that builds muscle mass, which causes their metabolism to run faster. So men can actually eat more calories than women do without gaining weight easily. Here are some tips that you should use to eat less when you're dining with friends or family:

1. Chew your food slowly.
2. Put your fork down between bites.
3. Stop eating when talking and resume eating slowly when conversation stops.
4. Don't be afraid to leave food on your plate.
5. If you're eating at home, when you feel full take your plate into the kitchen and return to the table. If there is no plate, there is no more food to pick at.

6.   Never order a meal to coincide with what your friends are ordering. Fatty, high-calorie meals sound good when someone else orders them; however, don't let their order be contagious.

7.   Don't try to keep up the pace with a fast eater at your table. They probably have no idea what or how much they are eating. They are usually talking a mile a minute while eating non-stop.

8.   Be careful of alcoholic beverages when dining with friends. Never order more than one drink if you do drink. If you're not a drinker, don't be afraid to not order a drink. Just get water or club soda with a twist. If you'd like a light drink, however, get a white wine spritzer (half the wine, half the calories, and club soda).

Dining out is difficult whether you are with company or whether you are alone. The reasons are that the portions are, at least, two to three times as large in restaurants as they would be at home. No one will give you a bad mark if you eat one-half of your meal and tell the waiter to wrap up the other half.

TIP # 78
FISH: THE BEST & THE WORST

Seafood is a good source of high-quality protein, nutrients and omega-3 fatty acids, which is an important part of a well-balanced healthful diet. Also, fish is a great diet food since it's low in calories and saturated fat, high in protein and contains the heart-protecting, cancer-fighting benefits of omega-3 fatty acids. Even though shellfish has higher levels of cholesterol than other types of fish, it is low in saturated fat and therefore does not raise your blood cholesterol.

It is important to realize that some fish are contaminated with high levels of methyl mercury. You can reduce your exposure to mercury by eating a variety of fish known to have low mercury levels. The FDA, however, recommends that women who are pregnant or nursing mothers limit their consumption of fish to 12 ounces of fish per week. The EPA suggests more stringent guidelines, limiting fish consumption in pregnant women or nursing mothers to one six-ounce meal of cooked fish per week and for young children to two ounces of cooked fish per week.

According to the FDA, the following fish are considered **The Best Fish** with the lowest levels of mercury:
1. Cod, catfish, crab, flounder, and sole
2. Grouper, haddock, herring, lobster, and mahi-mahi
3. Ocean perch, oysters, rainbow trout, and salmon
4. Sardines, scallops, tilapia, and farm-raised trout

The fish that contain the highest levels of mercury are considered **The Worst Fish** for human consumption. They are as follows:
1. Mackerel, shark, swordfish, and tile fish
2. Tuna—fresh or frozen
   a. Canned tuna, on the other hand, has lower levels of mercury, because the tuna used in the canning process are the smaller varieties of fish.

b. Canned tuna, labeled "chunk light" tuna has less mercury than "solid albacore" tuna.

You can reduce your exposure to mercury by eating those fish
listed as having lower levels of mercury. The health benefits of the nutrients contained in fish will, however, far outweigh the minimal exposure to
consuming fish with low levels of mercury. Also, be particularly careful
about taking fish-oil capsules, which may also contain high levels of mercury. Some better known, reliable companies are starting to list mercury
levels that are within the FDA's guidelines. These companies are endeav-
oring to use fish with low levels of mercury in their manufacturing process.
If no such listing is available on the label, then avoid that particular product.

TIP # 79
EAT ANYTHING YOU LIKE AND
STILL LOSE WEIGHT!

It isn't what you eat that makes you fat, it's actually how much or how many calories you eat that puts on weight. So, it's really not necessary to severely restrict your diet and deny yourself any of your favorite foods. If you just determine to eat less of the so-called forbidden foods, you'll be fine and you'll satisfy hunger cravings that ordinarily wouldn't be satisfied otherwise.

1.   Let's say you really like pasta, potatoes, or bread.

As long as you try to stay with the whole-wheat varieties, and in the case of potatoes, eat the skin or stick to a sweet potato, and you'll be fine. And better yet, if you add a serving of lean protein to a meal, which includes these forbidden bad carb foods, then the protein will actually decrease your craving for adding more of these so-called bad carbs to your meal. Protein is definitely more filling, so that you eat fewer calories with each meal than you would have eaten if you just were consuming fat or refined carbohydrates. Protein takes longer to digest and fills you up faster, while providing few calories and increased nutrition.

Research has shown that adding protein to each meal produces a higher body temperature and, therefore, a higher basal metabolic rate. This increases the number of calories burned in any 24-hour period. Protein-enriched meals take considerably longer to digest than carbohydrate meals, and therefore not only make you feel full earlier, but they contribute to a prolonged burning of calories, particularly fat stored in the body's fat cells. The result is more weight-loss when protein is added to each meal.

The Best Protein to add to bad carb meals includes lean meat and poultry, fish, peanut butter, nuts and legumes, low or nonfat milk, yogurt, and cheese, hard-boiled eggs, soy products, and sunflower or sesame seeds.

The Worst Protein includes marbled meats, hamburgers and cheeseburgers, high-fat dairy products, and processed meats. Bacon, sausage, and Canadian bacon are bad; however, a slice of extra lean ham has only 1 gram of fat and 38 calories.

2.   **Let's say that you have a sweet tooth and you can't get over a craving for cookies, cakes, ice cream, or candy.**

Have portable food handy whenever you go out (apple, orange, banana, pear, etc.) and munch on these when your sweet tooth surfaces. You're getting fewer calories and more fiber ounce for ounce from these healthy sweets.

If your appetite, however, goes into overdrive and you must have a forbidden sweet, then have it. Take one or two bites of the forbidden sweet and chew slowly, and then throw the rest of it away. Your sweet tooth will be satisfied and you will be minus the extra fat and calories.

Best Sweets: Fruits, nonfat jello or pudding with nonfat whipped cream, lightly sugared whole-grain cereal bites, non or low-fat ice cream (small amount because of high calorie content), low or nonfat yogurt, one slice of angel food cake with nonfat fudge, 1 Tbs., a smoothie (nonfat milk or yogurt blended with your favorite fruit), and diet soft drinks can also satisfy your sweet tooth.

Worst Sweets: Cakes, candy bars, sodas, cookies, doughnuts, pastries, candies, fruit juices without the fruit. Remember, if it really tastes good and sweet, you probably can't have it.

3.   Fat tastes good.

Let's face it – fat adds flavor to food and makes it taste good. Concentrate on eating the good fats, which actually taste as good as the bad fats.

a) For instance, instead of a cup of tuna salad with full-fat mayonnaise (20 grams of fat and 400 calories), use a small can of water-packed tuna with nonfat mayo (3 grams of fat and 225 calories) for your sandwich or salad.

b) Instead of bacon or sausage with your eggs, choose low-fat, lean ham (1 slice), which only has 1 gram of fat and 40 calories.

c) Instead of full-fat cream cheese on your bagel (scooped out, of course), use nonfat cream cheese and you save lots of fat and calories.

d) Also, low or nonfat cottage cheese tastes as good as the whole-fat variety, with a lot less calories and fat.

e) Substitute low or nonfat salad dressings or olive oil instead of full-fat salad dressings for your salads. Or, better yet, use lemon juice or flavored vinegars, with no calories at all.

f) Substitute two egg whites for whole eggs, and you'll save 80 calories and 10 grams of fat.

g) Instead of full-fat potato chips, make your own potato chips by slicing a small potato into thin slices and baking in the oven with olive oil vegetable spray. Add herbs if you'd like to vary the taste.

h) Substitute low-fat ice cream or low-fat yogurt instead of the whole-milk, whole-fat variety. The minimal fat content present in the low-fat yogurt and ice cream tastes just as good as the whole-fat variety.

i) Lean turkey or breast of chicken makes a nutritious, lean protein sandwich on whole-wheat bread with nonfat mayo.

Best Fats: Lean turkey or chicken, fish, lean cut meats (choose loin or round), nuts and legumes, peanut butter, low-fat dairy products, avocado, and canola and olive oils. Be sure to broil or grill all meats and fish and fowl.

Worst Fats: Fried foods, bread and butter, cream soups and sauces, whole-fat mayo and salad dressings, processed foods (crackers, cookies, and chips with trans fats), fatty, marbled meats, foods that are breaded, vegetables, meats, fish, and chicken that are saturated in butter or sauces, butter, margarine, and cooking oils, except for olive and canola oils.

4.   How cutting good carbs can be bad.

Complex high fiber carbohydrates (good carbs) are also necessary for the body to produce a natural anti-depressant hormone called **serotonin**. This hormone activates brain cells to produce a feeling of well being and calm, not unlike the endorphins which are hormones produced in the body as a result of exercise. Since women usually secrete less serotonin hormone than men, they naturally need more complex carbohydrates to produce this hormone.

If you reduce most carbohydrates, both refined and complex, from your meals as suggested by the typical low-carbohydrate diets, then your serotonin levels drop quickly, which results in a depressed, or "down" mood. This triggers a craving for all types of carbohydrates, particularly quick-acting refined carbohydrates (cakes, candies, pies, ice cream, etc.), which causes a rapid rise in blood sugar and serotonin levels, for a feeling of well-being. Unfortunately, this spike in serotonin is quickly aborted because the rapid rise in insulin levels causes both the blood sugar and serotonin levels to quickly abate. Now your mood plummets while your weight escalates.

Complex, high-fiber "good" carbs will keep your weight down and your mood high, by keeping your blood sugar and your serotonin levels elevated. Be thin! Be happy!

TIP # 80
FAT-FIGHTING FACTS

1. **Sneak in the veggies and the fruits.** Most people don't get their three servings each of fruits and vegetables daily. The way to sneak in your daily allotment of fruits and vegetables is to add them to most any food that you order or eat that doesn't come with fruits or vegetables included. For instance, get fruit (berries, bananas, apples) on your waffles or pancakes. Add green peppers, mushrooms, onions, broccoli, or spinach to your pizza. Put salsa on your salad or sandwich. Slice apples and pears and put grapes in your salads. Put a sliced banana on your peanut butter sandwich. Order a veggie burger instead of a meat burger. Load up any sandwich with cucumbers, tomatoes, lettuce, and sprouts.

2. **Dine at home more often.** The increase in obesity seems to coincide with the meals eaten out at restaurants, and not just fast-food restaurants. Skip the french fries, fried foods, cheeseburgers, sodas, and high-fat dressings for salads. Always choose grilled or baked foods without breading. Order hardy vegetable soup whenever possible and avoid cream soups. And, most importantly, don't finish those oversized meals that most restaurants put in front of you. Eat one-half the meal and take the other half home, or give it away.

3. **Eat more frequently.** Small frequent meals keep your body fueled throughout the day and prevent you from overeating at any particular time of day or night. Small meals with lean protein and high fiber added keep your appetite satisfied for hours without any hunger pangs. Adding the lean protein to these small, frequent meals increases your energy

level. If you skip breakfast or lunch, your metabolism slows down, causing a spike in insulin levels when you finally eat. This makes it harder for your body to burn fat efficiently. The result: weight gain, not weight-loss. This type of small, frequent meal eating helps you to condition yourself to keeping portion sizes small when you eat at home or at a restaurant.

4.   **Don't skip breakfast.** Studies have proved that people who eat a healthy breakfast every day are the most successful dieters. Healthy breakfasts of whole-grain, high-fiber cereal topped with fruit and skim milk is a great way to start the day, or an egg fried in a small amount of olive oil on a slice of toasted whole-wheat bread makes a great lean protein start for your day. A slice of whole-wheat bread topped with a Tbs. of all-fruit jelly and/or peanut butter is an appetite-satisfying breakfast. People who regularly eat a healthy breakfast don't get hungry for midmorning snacks of doughnuts or muffins. Your body's appetite control mechanism stays in check for long periods of time, without any spikes in blood sugar or blood insulin levels. And besides, a nutritious breakfast causes your body to burn fat more efficiently and starts your diet-day off perfectly.

5.   **Always check the labels when buying food.** See how many calories are in a serving size and also check how many servings are in the entire package that you are considering purchasing. Make sure that the saturated fat and the sugar contents are low. The first listed ingredient on the ingredients label is the one that is the highest concentration in the food that you are buying. If sugars or fats are listed first, then put it back on the shelf.

6.   **Be careful of soft drinks.** Sweetened soft drinks contain loads of sugar and calories. In addition to sodas, this includes sweetened iced teas, fat-loaded calories in coffee

drinks, such as lattes and cappuccinos, and juices that contain little or no juice, but lots of sugar. Stay away from so-called energy drinks, which contain high amounts of sugar and caffeine. These drinks are unhealthy and the energy that they produce initially is from the initial shot of caffeine and glucose absorbed into the bloodstream. These drinks cause unhealthy spikes in both blood sugar and blood insulin, and the high caffeine content of these drinks can be dehydrating. Be sure to choose diet sodas and teas. Switch to fat-free coffee drinks without sugar, cream or whole milk. Choose 100% fruit juices and 100% vegetable juices. Drink lots of water, seltzer, and fat-free milk.

7. **Eat Less.** To lose weight, you have got to eat less. People have a tendency to clean their plates, no matter how large the portion size is. Most restaurant portions are more than twice the serving size at home, so share it with a companion or take the other half home, or you can order two appetizers instead of an entrée. Avoid oversized bowls and plates at home, which tend to hold larger portions. Concentrate on smaller servings and pause during a meal to give your appetite control mechanism time to let you know that you're actually full, and be careful not to eat fast, because you will consume mass quantities of calories before you'll ever know that you're not hungry any longer.

8. **Exercise to burn more calories than you eat.** It's not necessary to join a gym or participate in aerobics classes to burn up fat. You can burn calories by just climbing the stairs, cleaning the house, riding a bike, working in the garden, or just by walking 30 minutes every day. You don't even have to work up a sweat to burn calories while exercising. Studies have proven that people who take a brisk walk for 30 minutes every day burn body fat, improve their physical fitness, and lower their blood pressure,

as much as, if not even more than, people who work out at a gym three to four days per week. Even two 15-minute walks per day will give you the same fitness and fat-burning benefits as a 30-minute walk every day. A recent study from a major university showed that sedentary women, in addition to gaining weight in their abdomens, buttocks, and thighs, actually increased their deep fat that surrounds the internal organs of the body. This increases the risk of heart disease, hypertension, and diabetes. The study also showed that moderate exercise five times per week for 30 to 40 minutes decreased the deep fat by more than 35% and resulted in considerable weight-loss over a three-month period.

TIP # 81
ANTIOXIDANTS & EXERCISE

Among the many health claims regarding antioxidant supplements, there has been little discussion in the way that the body itself actually combats damage caused by *free radicals*. Living cells have evolved a variety of internal systems that offer protection against oxidative stress (the term commonly used to describe free-radical attack). Oxidative stress is an imbalance between the factors that cause oxidation and the factors that inhibit oxidation. The basic cause of oxidative stress is the formation of free-radicals. Free radicals are the culprits that make the body's metabolic system and the organs' systems break down. It is important to understand how the body protects itself against free radical attacks.

There are may selected antioxidant nutrients that are found in primary food sources; for example, fresh fruits and vegetables, grains and oils, yeast, and many other food groups. The nutrients range from vitamin C, vitamin E, carotenoids, coenzyme Q10, glutathione, and many other phytonutrients, vitamins, and minerals. Here is a surprising addition to the list of agents that affect the body's oxidation process: regular exercise can influence the equilibrium between antioxidation and oxidation, or the oxidative balance. In other words, *regular exercise acts as an antioxidant* just like any dietary or food supplement, helping the body to rid itself of free radicals.

The following is an interesting comparison of the different types of physical exercise when studied at the molecular level. Physical activity influences oxidative balance, but it does so paradoxically. During acute phases of physical activity, for example, strenuous exercise, more oxygen is needed to create energy; therefore, more volatile oxygen molecules are formed. During this type of strenuous exercise, highly reactive hydroxyl radicals can overwhelm the body's antioxidant systems, and cause injury to the surrounding cells and tissues. Hence, **isolated strenuous exercise produces significant oxidative stress**. However, when physical activity is recurrent or moderate (for example, a walking program), exercise-induced oxidative stress decreases over time, as the internal antioxidant systems begin to adapt. Thus, **regular exercise improves oxidative balance**. This is a very complicated way of stating, on a molecular level, what we have been stating all along, that *strenuous exercise can be hazardous to your health, whereas regular exercise, like walking, is beneficial to your health.*

Regular aerobic exercise, such as walking, may improve the oxidative balance in several ways. One way is that it improves the antioxidant protection by regulating enzyme systems that are responsible for cleaning up escaped free radicals. Secondly, it probably decreases resting levels of free radical formation. To put it another way, sedentary people tend to have poor oxidative balance because they undergo oxidative stress even at relatively low levels of physical functioning, whereas fit people tend to have good oxidative balance, because they limit oxidative stress during exercise and during daily functioning. So, the next time you remember to take your dietary antioxidant, whether in food or supplement form, remember to continue your walking exercise program to obtain additional antioxidant protection against those nasty free radicals. The result is that you'll look younger and live longer. And you'll lose considerable weight without any change whatsoever in your diet.

TIP # 82
BURN CALORIES & GET FIRM!

FIGURE CONTROL

Your body burns calories all the time **(basal metabolic rate)** no matter what you are doing. Even when you are sleeping, between 50 and 85 calories an hour are expended during that time. This is why it takes a certain amount of dietary calories daily just to maintain your body weight. Therefore, it is obvious that if you are actually doing something in the form of a physical activity like a walking exercise program, you will burn up more calories than your normal basal metabolic rate, which only involves sedentary activities like sleeping, eating, and sitting.

Remember that with **walking**, you increase the **aerobic capacity**, which is the body's ability to take in more oxygen through the lungs, dissolve it into the bloodstream, and pump it more efficiently, so that it circulates to all of the muscles and cells of the body. This oxygen is used to produce energy. As this oxygen burns off fat, you will have a trimmer, leaner figure.

As surprising as it sounds, walking is the most reliable and safe way to lose excess fat and flab. Crash diets and fad diets may do a faster job, but they usually are dangerous, exhausting, monotonous, and debilitating. It is also a known fact that people who take off weight on rapid weight reduction programs put the weight back on just as fast as they took it off. Weight reduction through walking is a more gradual process, and the most important point to note is, that the chances of regaining back the weight is minimal. This is because the body has gone through a time-consuming metabolic process, in which the adjustment to the weight-loss and weight maintenance has been gradual. Subsequently, no rapid weight gain has been noted in people who have been on a continuous walking program.

HOW FAR DO YOU HAVE TO WALK?

One of the most important things that you have to be aware of is, that in order to begin a walking exercise program, you do not have to be an exercise fanatic. You do not have to be a jogger or an aerobic exercise junkie to accrue the benefits of an aerobic exercise-walking program. You will see that there are many ways to augment your walking program by walking at particular times of the day or evening when you would ordinarily ride in your car. For example, when you are driving or taking the bus to work, park or get off the bus a few blocks from your place of employment, and walk that short distance. For lunch, you can take a half-hour walk out of your lunch break and enjoy the fresh air. Also, at work you can concentrate on using the stairs more often, instead of using the elevator.

Many people think that because they are active all day at home or in the office, that they are actually getting enough exercise. Nothing could be further from the truth. You are not expending the number of calories that are needed in a weight reduction or weight maintenance program by these activities. There is no doubt that you are expending some energy, but you will need to supplement this with your **regular walking program**.

ON A CLEAR DAY YOU CAN WALK FOREVER

Most of us do not realize that we walk more than **125,000 miles in an average lifetime**. Walking is a complex physiological and biomechanical process of getting from one place to another. Walking involves using hundreds of muscles, thousands of nerves, and many bones, joints, and ligaments to produce a near-perfect biomechanical method of walking, which involves the synchronous movement of the legs and arms.

The **rhythm** of walking involves walking at a steady pace, which will become automatic, and the brain will regulate the length of your stride, your heart rate, oxygen uptake, and the other physiological adjustments. You should concentrate on making smooth, even steps, avoiding spurts of speed and abrupt changes in pace. The energy expenditure over your walking period will remain constant, and your walk should leave you feeling completely relaxed, with an effortless motion. Colon Fletcher, author of The Complete Walker, said it best when referring to rhythm; "An easy, unbroken rhythm can carry you along hour after hour, almost without your being aware that you are putting one foot in front of the other."

The **speed** of walking should be between 2.5 and 3.5 miles per hour, since walking is a moderate-type of aerobic exercise. If you increase your speed beyond 4 miles per hour, the upper arms and shoulders swing too fast, and the lower leg muscles have to work too hard to compensate, thus producing wasteful energy expenditure. It is important that you walk at a comfortable speed, one that does not leave you breathless. This type of walking activity falls into the **aerobic** form of exercise, in which you are taking in **oxygen** as fast as you are burning it up. This is termed the efficient use of energy. **Anaerobic** exercise, on the other hand, is the opposite condition, which is caused by an overexertion of muscles (For example: running fast, lifting heavy weights, etc.) working beyond their capacity. This type of anaerobic exercise leads to the buildup of **lactic acid** in the muscles, causing pain, discomfort, and fatigue, a condition known as **oxygen debt**.

The **gait** of walking refers to the motions of your legs, feet, and arms during the phases of walking. The muscles and joints of the ankles, knees, and hips provide most of the energy required for walking. When we over-stride or under-stride, we disrupt the natural walking gait. An easy, steady, unbroken stride will produce the rhythm and gait necessary for the effortless act of walking. Also, it is necessary to avoid toeing in or toeing out during the walking gait, since this wastes energy. Try to concentrate on keeping your toes straight, and thus your stride will be even and rhythmic. During the act of walking, your arms swing naturally from the shoulders. Over-swinging the arms purposely during walking will reduce the efficiency of the act of walking and subsequently tire you out early during your walk. If you don't try to concentrate on the act of walking during your rhythmic stride, you will actually allow the muscles to relax and perform more efficiently.

TIPS ON BUYING WALKING SHOES

1. Always buy a good pair of walking shoes. Make sure the shoes fit properly. Don't choose shoes by their size. Choose them by how they fit on your feet. Remember, sizes vary among different shoe brands and styles.

2. The size of your feet changes, as you grow older. It is a good idea to have your foot size re-measured before buying new shoes. In most people, one foot is larger than the other. When you go shoe shopping, have both feet measured. Then select shoes that fit the largest foot.

3. Try to find shoes that conform as closely as possible to the shape of your foot.

4. If possible, try on shoes at the end of the day. That's when your feet are at their largest and widest.

5. Stand up when you are trying on shoes. Make sure there is enough space between the end of the shoe and your longest toe. Shoes should be at least ½ to ¾ of an inch longer than your longest toe. The toe section should be wide and high enough so as not to cause compression of your toes.

6. Make sure the ball of your foot fits comfortably into the widest part of your shoe. And there should be enough cushioning material to make your foot feel comfortable and springy.

7. Don't buy shoes that feel tight, hoping they will stretch.

8. Select shoes that fit your heel comfortably and allow a minimum amount of slippage.

9. The sole and heel should be made of a thick, resilient material that absorbs the shock of walking on a hard surface.

10. And above all, make sure the shoes feel comfortable. Walk in the shoes that you want to buy to make sure that they fit and feel right.

IX.
DIET-STEP® TIPS

TIP # 83
WALK OFF WEIGHT!

Women are more likely to perceive themselves as fat, whereas in reality, men are more likely to be overweight. In a recent Harris poll of over 1,200 women and men nationwide, the findings were as follows:

* Over 50% of women considered themselves overweight, compared to 38% of men.
* 65% of the men were actually overweight, compared with 62% of the woman.
* Almost 40% of those people surveyed stated that they were on a diet.
* 60% of those surveyed were overweight, which was exactly the same percentage as last year's survey.
* More than 50% of those surveyed felt they weren't getting enough exercise.

It doesn't appear that we're getting any thinner despite all of the diet books, health clubs, fitness centers, and diet promoters! So what's the answer? Walking, of course! Walkers, by and large, are the least overweight segment of any population group. This fact has been verified in numerous medical studies.

"I DON'T REALLY EAT THAT MUCH!"

The question I get asked most often from patients about being overweight is, "How come I keep gaining weight? I don't really eat that much." Well, the truth of the matter is that we get heavier as we get older because our physical activity tends to decrease even though our food intake stays the same. The only way to beat the battle of the bulge is to burn those unwanted pounds away. Walking actually **burns calories**. The following table will give you an idea as to the energy expended in walking, which is actually the number of calories burned per minute or per hour, by walking at different speeds.

TABLE I

WALKING SPEED	CALORIES BURNED/ MINUTE	CALORIES BURNED/ 30 MINUTES	CALORIES BURNED/ HOUR
Slow Speed (2 mph)	4-5	130-160	260-320
Brisk Speed (3 mph)	5-6	160-190	320-380
Fast Speed (4 mph)	6-7	190-220	380-440
Race Walking (5 mph)	7-8	220-260	440-520

A pound of body fat contains approximately 3,500 calories. When you eat 3,500 more calories than your body actually needs, it stores up that pound as body fat. If you reduce your intake by 3,500 calories, you will lose a pound. It doesn't make any difference how long it takes your body to store or burn these 3,500 calories. The result is always the same. You either gain or lose one pound of body fat, depending on how long it takes you to accumulate or burn up 3,500 calories.

You can then actually lose weight by just walking. When you walk at a speed of 3 mph for *one hour every day*, you will burn up *350 calories each day*. Therefore, if you walk *one hour a day for ten days*, then you will burn up to a total of *3,500 calories*. Since there are 3,500 calories in each pound of fat, when you burn up 3,500 calories by walking, you will lose a pound of body fat. You will continue to lose one pound of body fat every time you complete ten hours of walking at a speed of 3 mph. **It works every time!**

If you just count calories, your chances of losing weight are minimal. *Walking,* however, is a certain way towards permanent weight reduction. The majority of obese people are much less active than the majority of thin people. It is their sedentary lifestyle that accounts for their excess weight and not their overeating. If they just took a brisk walk for one hour every day, they could lose 18 pounds in six months, or 36 pounds in one year, without any change in their diets.

If you want to lose weight permanently, then the energy burned during your exercise should come from **fats** and not from carbohydrates. During the first 20 to 30 minutes of moderate exercise like walking, only one-third of the energy burned comes from carbohydrates, whereas two-thirds comes from body fats. During short bursts of exercise, two-thirds of the energy burned comes from carbohydrates and only one-third from body fat. It stands to reason, then, that a continuous exercise, like walking, which burns primarily body fats, is a lot better for permanent weight reduction than short spurts of strenuous exercise (examples: jogging, calisthenics, racquetball, etc.).

If you increase the duration of your daily walking from 20 minutes to 30-60 minutes, you will burn more energy from body fats, resulting in faster weight-loss. Once you've lost your weight, you will maintain your weight better by walking *20-30 minutes every day* than by doing calisthenics, raquet-ball, jogging, etc. for 15 to 20 minutes. This occurs because you will be burning a higher proportion of body fats rather than by just burning carbohydrates.

Strenuous exercise after a large meal causes the increased blood supply in the stomach and intestinal tract to be diverted to the exercising muscles. This puts a strain on the cardiovascular system, especially in anyone who has a heart or circulatory problem. A calm *walk*, on the other hand, approximately 45 to 60 minutes after eating, does not stress the cardiovascular system and burns many of the excess calories that you should not have eaten in the first place. It's far better to get up and walk away from that big meal before you overstuff your face. When you physically walk away from the table, you are removing yourself from temptation, but even more importantly, you are allowing the fullness control center in your brain to catch up to what's really going on in your stomach. You are actually full, but you don't know it yet. I always tell my patients that, *"eating less and walking more"* are the only two ways to lose weight effectively, or, to put it another way – *"walk more and eat less!"*

Many studies have clearly documented the **weight-loss effects of exercise**. Even more important is that the weight-loss caused by walking is almost all due to the ***burning of body fat***, not carbohydrates. This weight-loss or weight maintenance can be continued indefinitely as long as you walk regularly. You are literally **Walking Off Weight** .

Walking *before meals* decreases your appetite; in addition, recent studies show that walking approximately 45 to 60 minutes *after eating* increases the metabolic body rate to burn away calories at a faster rate. It appears, then, that walking after eating is another way to lose additional pounds. Never walk, however, immediately after a large meal is ingested, which you shouldn't have eaten in the first place.

This burning of calories at a faster rate has been explained as a combination of the energy expended from walking and the calories burned from the actual ingestion of food itself. This is called the ***Thermic Effect of Food*** or the ***Specific Dynamic Action***. We actually burn more calories as we eat because the energy metabolism of the body actually increases 5-10%. This doesn't mean that the more you eat, the more calories you'll burn. But it is a good reason for *walking 45-60 minutes after small meals* for additional weight-loss. If you want to lose weight at a faster rate, then walk before meals to cut down your appetite and walk approximately 45 to 60 minutes after small meals to burn more calories. ***W.O.W.! (Walking Off Weight)– What an easy way to diet!***

TIP # 84
WON'T EXERCISE MAKE YOU HUNGRY?

Another myth regarding diet and exercise is that exercise stimulates the appetite. So, after exercise, you're hungry, you eat more, and you cancel out any calories you burned during exercise. Right? **Wrong!**

Contrary to popular belief, walking actually decreases your appetite. It does this by several mechanisms, which are described as follows:

1.   **Walking regulates the brain's appetite control center** (appestat), which controls your hunger pangs. Too little exercise causes your appetite to increase by stimulating the appestat to make you hungry. Walking, on the other hand, slows the appestat down, thus decreasing your hunger pangs.

2.   **Walking redirects the blood supply away from your stomach**, towards the exercising muscles. With less blood supplied to the stomach, your appetite is reduced.

3.   **Walking burns fat rather than carbohydrates**, and therefore does not drop the blood sugar precipitously. Strenuous exercises and very low calorie diets both drop the blood sugar rapidly, and it is this low blood sugar that stimulates your appetite and makes you hungry. Walking, on the other hand, is a more moderate type of exercise and consequently burns fats slowly, rather than carbohydrates quickly. This results in the blood sugar remaining constant. And when the blood sugar remains level, you do not feel hungry.

4.   **Walking also helps to increase the resting basal metabolic rate (BMR).** This basal metabolic rate refers to the calories your body burns at rest in order to produce energy. When you go on a calorie-restriction diet, your BMR slows down. This is because your body assumes that the reduction in calories is the result of starvation, and your body wants to burn fewer calories so that you won't starve to death. The body has no way of knowing that you're on a diet. This is

also one of the reasons that you don't continue to lose weight on a calorie restriction diet. The body prevents this excess weight-loss by lowering its BMR, so that you stop losing weight, even though you are eating the same number of calories that you ate in the beginning of your diet.

If, however, you are combining walking with your diet, then the walking keeps the BMR elevated even though you are dieting. So, in effect, it prevents the BMR from dropping and burning fewer calories, as when you are dieting alone. The result: Less hunger and more calories burned when you walk every day.

TIP # 85
20 MINUTES A DAY MELTS
POUNDS AWAY

With the advent of the computer age, people are forced by design to do less and less physical labor. It would seem logical that this would result in more energy being available for other activities. However, how many times have you noticed that the less you do, the more tired you feel, whereas the more active you are, the more energy you have for other activities? Exercise improves the efficiency of the lungs, the heart, and the circulatory system in their ability to take in and deliver *oxygen* throughout the entire body. This oxygen is the catalyst which burns the fuel (food) we take in to produce energy. Consequently, the more oxygen we take in, the more *energy* we have for all of our activities.

Oxygen is the vital ingredient that is necessary for our survival. Since oxygen can't be stored, our cells need a continuous supply in order to remain healthy. Walking increases your body's ability to extract oxygen from the air, so that increased amounts of oxygen are available for every organ, tissue, and cell in the body. Walking actually increases the *total volume* of blood, making more red blood cells available to carry oxygen and nutrition to the tissues, and to remove carbon dioxide and waste products from the body's cells. This increased saturation of the tissues with oxygen is also aided by the opening of *small blood vessels*, which is another direct result of walking.

So let's take that first step for energy, fitness, and real weight-loss. Walking every day will keep a fresh supply of oxygen surging through your blood vessels to all of your body's hungry cells. Don't disappoint these little fellows, because you depend on them as much as they depend on you. If you shortchange them on their daily oxygen supply, they'll take it out on you in the form of illness and disease.

20 MINUTE DIET-STEP® WALKING PLAN

Twenty minutes of walking every day except Sunday is all that you need to complete the Diet-Step Walking Plan. Either 20 minutes outdoors (walking) or 20 minutes indoors (stationary bike or treadmill) will provide you with maximum cardiovascular fitness, good health, and boundless energy. Remember, this 20-minute walk is a basic part of your weight-loss program in the Diet-Step Walking Plan. The 20-minute walk, six days per week, is what burns the extra calories needed to lose weight and to decrease your appetite when you're on a regular walking program. This walking plan also provides the fuel that powers your energy level throughout your day.

When you first start your walking program, pick a level terrain, since hills place too much strain and stress on your legs, hips, and back muscles. Concentrate on maintaining *erect posture* while walking and every so often contract your abdominal muscles to strengthen your abs. Walk with your shoulders relaxed and your arms carried in a relatively low position, with natural motion at the elbow. Don't hold your arms too high when you walk; otherwise, you will develop muscle spasms and pain in your neck, back, and shoulder muscles.

Make sure you walk at a *brisk pace* (approximately 3 to 3.5 mph) for maximum efficiency. When you begin walking, your respiration and heart rate will automatically become faster; however, if you feel short of breath or tired, then you're probably walking too fast. Remember to stop whenever you are tired or fatigued, and then resume walking after resting. Concentrate on walking naturally, putting *energy* into each step. Soon you will begin to feel relaxed and comfortable as your stride becomes smooth and effortless. Walk with an even *steady* gait and your own rhythm of walking will automatically develop into an unconscious synchronous movement.

ONLY 4 WEEKS TO LOSE 6-8 POUNDS

Your walking program should be planned to meet your individual schedule; however, when you begin walking, it's a good idea to walk at a specific time every day to ensure regularity and consistency. You will be able to vary your schedule once you have started the program. Lunchtime, for example, is an ideal time to plan a 20-minute walk, since it combines both calorie burning and calorie reduction. If you have less time for lunch, you'll eat less.

Gradually build up your six-day-per-week walking times. The first week, walk *5 minutes* daily, six days per week. The second week, walk *10 minutes* six days per week. The third week, walk *15 minutes* per day. And finally, by the fourth week, start to walk *20 minutes* every day, six days per week. Remember, the speed of walking is not important, unless you are walking too slowly (under 2 mph). The most important factor is that you walk regularly at a relatively brisk pace. If you become tired easily, or get short of breath or develop pain anywhere, or if any other unusual symptoms occur, check with your physician immediately.

The Diet-Step® walking method is the ideal weight control and fitness program. Studies in human physiology have proven that walking acts as a weight reduction plan without actually dieting and as a fitness program without strenuous exercises. Too often today, we allow a sedentary lifestyle to dominate our daily living. We sit at our desks all day and in front of the TV set in the evenings. We drive to our destination, no matter how close or how far, instead of doing what's easy, natural, and healthful – walking.

Most of us would rather spend 15 minutes in our cars waiting at the drive-in window of a bank, rather than getting out and walking the length of the parking lot. Even at work, we opt for the elevator, even if it's only for a few floors. At the supermarket or shopping mall, most of us would rather drive around the parking lot several times, so that we can get a parking spot closer to the store. These are all good opportunities to do the Diet-Step®, not the car-step. Use your feet, not your wheels, and you'll look great and feel full of pep when you do the Diet-Step®.

Remember, it's the amount of *TIME* that you walk every day that is more important than the distance, or even the speed. If you walk *20 minutes every day*, it doesn't make any difference whether you are walking 2.5, 3, 3.5, or 4 miles per hour. You are still burning calories, losing weight, and developing physical fitness. In other words, it doesn't matter how far you walk or how fast you walk, as long as you walk regularly. *You'll be walking six days each week to lose weight, keep fit and boost energy.*

Once you've started walking six days per week, you will begin to notice the many changes brought about by your improved aerobic fitness and maximum oxygen capacity (the uptake and distribution of oxygen through your body). You will have lots of pep and energy, a trim figure, improved breathing capacity and muscle tone, improved exercise tolerance, a better night's sleep, a feeling of peace and relaxation, and a lessening of tension. Once you have completed this four-week conditioning program, you will have taken the first steps towards improved cardiovascular fitness, good health, and a long, happy life. Then, all you need to do is walk 20 minutes every day except Sunday to reap all of the fitness benefits of the Diet-Step® Plan.

The great part about walking as an exercise is that you aren't limited to a particular time or location. Walking doesn't require special clothes or equipment. You can walk before or after work, or if you drive to work, you can park your car a block or two from the office and walk the rest of the way. If you take the bus or train, get off a stop before your station and walk. An enclosed mall could be the perfect place for your walk in bad weather. Remember to take 20 minutes from your lunch break and walk. Just think of how good that fresh air will feel and smell.

TIP # 86
FASTER WEIGHT-LOSS WALKING PLANS

The **DIET-STEP® WALKING PROGRAM** is based on walking at a brisk pace (3 mph) – without any change whatsoever in your diet. This weight-loss program is based upon calories *burned by walking only*. In order to increase the amount of weight that you can lose by walking, you will have to increase the number of minutes that you walk every day. This faster weight-loss occurs because you will be walking for more than just the 20 minutes, six days per week, as on the 20-MinuteDiet-Step® Walking Plan.

Three miles per hour is a speed that can be maintained for a long duration without causing stress, strain, or fatigue. We are not talking about window-shopping walking, which is much too slow (1 to 2 mph), and which is not at all useful in burning calories. Nor are we suggesting fast walking (4 to 5 mph), which is too fast to be continued for long periods of time without tiring. And we certainly are not recommending race walking (5 to 6 mph), which is worthless as a permanent weight reduction plan, and has all of the same hazards and dangers that jogging or strenuous exercises have.

The following walking plans have been designed for *faster weight-loss* than the weight-loss on the regular 20 Minute Diet-Step® Plan. You can walk anywhere, anytime, anyplace, as long as you make the time. Remember, you can always take the time to fit a walk into your schedule. And if you don't have the time – make it! Don't *wait to lose weight*, when just walking will make your *figure look great.*

DIET-STEP® WALKING-OFF-WEIGHT PLANS

1. DIET-STEP® PLAN #1: (LOSE ONE ADDITIONAL POUND EVERY 20 DAYS)

On this Diet-Step® plan, you will walk for **one hour every other day** or **one-half hour every day**. Walking at a brisk 3 mph pace, you will burn approximately **350 calories every hour that you walk**. Let's see how much weight you'll lose by this plan.

1.   Walk ½ hour daily x 350 calories/hour = 174 calories burned per day.
2.   Walk 3 ½ hours per week x 350 calories/hour = 1,225 calories burned per week.
3.   Walk 10 hours every 20 days x 350 calories/hour = 3,500 calories burned or one pound lost every 20 days (or 175 calories burned per day x 20 days = 3,500 calories).
4.   On this Walking-Off-Weight Diet-Step® plan, you will lose **one additional pound every 20 days, or 1 ½ pounds every month**.

2.   DIET-STEP® PLAN #2: (LOSE ONE ADDITIONAL POUND EVERY 10 DAYS)

On this Diet-Step® plan, you can lose **one additional pound every 10 days** just walking **one hour every day of the week**. The only difference in this plan is that you are now walking an hour every day. You will still be burning up 350 calories every hour that you walk briskly (3 mph).

Remember, this Diet-Step® plan also works without any change in your current diet plan. Since it takes 10 hours of walking at 3 mph to burn up 3,500 calories or one pound, if you walk for an hour every day, you will lose **one additional pound every 10 days**. By following this plan, you can actually lose an additional **3 extra pounds every month**.

3.   DIET-STEP® PLAN #3: (LOSE ONE ADDITIONAL POUND EVERY WEEK)

For those of you who want to lose weight even faster, you can walk for **45 minutes twice daily**. By walking a total of **1 ½ hours every day** of the week, you will be able to speed up the Walking-Off-Weight Diet-Step® plan. When you walk 1 ½ hours every day, you will burn up 525 calories each day or 3,675 calories per week. You can see that you will lose a pound a week on this plan, with a few extra (175) calories to spare. You may divide your 1 ½ hours of walking into **three 30-minute** sessions daily if that's more convenient for you. The weight loss results will be the same. This plan will enable you to lose one **additional pound every week**, or about **4 extra pounds a month**.

Again, all this additional weight-loss occurs without your changing one thing in your Diet-Step® plan. By following any one of these three accelerated Diet-Step® walking plans, you will be able to lose more weight than you can lose on the regular 20-Minute Diet-Step® plan alone. *Remember, it's easy to lose weight and look your best. Just do the Diet-Step®.*

TIP # 87
DIET-STEP® CHEATER'S PLAN

Let's say your weight is just where you'd like it to be, but you don't want to gain another ounce. Or say your weight is nowhere near what you would like it to be, but you really can't afford to gain another pound without going into another dress size. Each of you would like to be able to cheat and at least stay the same weight. Well, fear no more, **DIET-STEP® CHEATER'S PLAN** is just for you.

How about a piece of candy, a slice of cake, french fries, a cone of ice cream, a slice of pizza, or a glass of wine? With the **DIET-STEP® CHEATER'S PLAN**, you have the perfect method that allows you to cheat without paying the price. Eat your favorite snack food, consult the following table **(TABLE II)**, and walk the number of minutes listed in order to burn up the extra calories you've cheated on. The following table shows how many minutes of walking at a brisk pace (3 mph) are necessary to burn up the caloric value of those foods listed.

If your favorite snack food is not listed on the following table, you can easily figure out the time you have to burn off your snack's calories. Look up the number of calories of your favorite snack food and divide by the number 6. This answer will give you the number of minutes it takes to walk off your snack. The number 6 comes from the fact that walking at a brisk pace (3 mph) burns approximately 6 calories per minute. Example: frankfurter and roll = 300 calories. Divide 6 into 300 and you get 50. It will take you 50 minutes to walk off this snack. "Hot Dog!"

TABLE II

DIET-STEP® CHEATER'S PLAN
BRISK WALKING (3 MPH) BURNS SNACKS

American cheese (1 slice)	16 minutes

Apple (medium)	15 minutes
Apple juice (6 ounces)	17 minutes
Bagel (1)	23 minutes
Banana (medium)	16 minutes
Beer (12 ounces)	30 minutes
Bologna sandwich	50 minutes
Candy bar (1 ounce)	45 minutes
Cake (1 slice pound cake)	63 minutes
Chocolate bar/nuts (1 ounce)	28 minutes
Cheese crackers (6)	35 minutes
Cheese steak (1/2)	55 minutes
Chicken, fried (3 pieces)	50 minutes
Chocolate cookies (3)	25 minutes
Corn chips (small pack)	33 minutes
Doughnut (jelly)	40 minutes
Frankfurter & roll	50 minutes
French fries (3 ounces)	50 minutes
Hamburger (4 ounces) & roll	73 minutes
Ice cream cone	30 minutes
Ice cream sundae	75 minutes
Milk shake, chocolate (8 ounces)	42 minutes
Muffin, blueberry	25 minutes
Orange juice (6 ounces)	16 minutes
Peanut butter crackers (6)	50 minutes
Peanuts, in shell (2 ounces)	37 minutes
Pie, apple (1 slice)	46 minutes
Pizza (1 slice)	40 minutes
Potato chips (small pack)	33 minutes
Pretzels (hard – 3 small)	30 minutes
Pretzels (soft – 1 Superpretzel®)	30 minutes
Shrimp cocktail (6 small)	18 minutes
Soda – cola (12 ounces)	24 minutes
Tuna fish sandwich	41 minutes
Wine, Chablis (4 ounces)	14 minutes
Whiskey, rye (1 ounce)	17 minutes

TIP # 88
WALKERS WIN BY STAYING THIN!

The question always comes up as to when you should exercise. Is it before or after eating? How long before? How long after? Many professional athletes schedule their day's activities around their meals. Also, many fitness enthusiasts actually become fanatical and inflexible about the time sequence of exercise and meals. Although walkers don't have to be as particular about timing their walking in relation to mealtime, it's still essential to become familiar, at least in part, with the physiology of digestion.

As food enters your stomach, the heart pumps a significant quantity of blood into the stomach to aid digestion. This does not pose a problem when you are at rest, but if you decide to exercise immediately after eating, then there is a conflict of interests. The stomach now has to compete with the exercising muscles for the blood it needs for digestion. If the exercise gets vigorous, then digestion is arrested and you begin to feel bloated and develop abdominal cramps. Exercise should, therefore, begin after a meal has passed through the stomach and small intestines. This takes approximately two to three hours after ingesting a large meal, and from 60 to 90 minutes after eating a smaller meal.

Foods high in fat and protein are digested slowly and tend to remain in the digestive tract for a longer time than a meal that is higher in complex carbohydrates (vegetables, fruits, whole-grain cereals, and whole-grain breads and pasta). Foods that are high in refined sugar, like cakes, candy, and pies, can trigger an excess insulin response if they are eaten immediately before exercise. This means that the excess insulin produced as a result of the high sugar content of food, combined with the exertion of exercise, could drop your blood sugar rapidly. This could result in weakness, muscle cramps, and even fainting.

On the other hand, fasting for long periods prior to exercise is, in itself, counter-productive. In order to replenish the stores of liver and muscle glycogen needed for energy, it is necessary to eat several hours before exercising. With fasting, you are depleting these energy stores, and exercise then becomes difficult and tiring without adequate fuel storage reserves for energy.

So what does this all have to do with walking and eating? Very little, if anything. Most of these rules of digestion apply to strenuous and vigorous exercise with relation to mealtime. They do, however, affect us somewhat with regard to our walking program. The most important fact to be learned from this discussion on digestive physiology is that it is essential that you don't walk immediately after eating, especially if you've consumed a relatively large meal (which you shouldn't be eating in the first place). This puts a strain on the cardiovascular system and can even deprive the heart of its own essential blood supply, particularly if you exercise vigorously immediately after eating (which you shouldn't be doing in the second place).

Walking, however, 45 to 60 minutes after a small meal and 60 to 90 minutes after a moderate meal, can actually aid in digestion by nudging the foodstuffs gently along the digestive tract. This in no way competes for the blood in the digestive tract, since the walking muscles do not pig-out for every available ounce of oxygen like the strenuously exercising muscle-gluttons. In fact, the gentle art of walking allows oxygen to be evenly distributed to all of the body's internal organs, which, in this particular case, is the digestive tract.

Recent studies indicate a four-fold advantage for dieters who walk before and after meals. As we have previously seen, walking before eating quiets down our appetite control center in the brain and makes us less hungry. Secondly, walking at any time burns calories directly, as we walk. And thirdly, new studies in exercise physiology have shown that walking anywhere from 45 to 90 minutes after eating a small to moderate-sized meal will actually burn 10-15% more calories than walking on an empty stomach. This is explained by a term called the *thermic dynamic action of food.* What this means is that the actual digestion of foodstuffs, combined with the gentle action of walking, results in a slightly higher metabolic rate, thus burning more calories per hour. And lastly, newer research has indicated that you continue to burn calories long after you complete your walking exercise program. Four great reasons to keep walking for weight-loss and weight-maintenance.

TIP # 89
HOW TO GET BACK INTO
YOUR CLOTHES

BEAUTY BENEFITS OF WALKING

Every time you start out on your daily walk, literally thousands of changes occur in your body. Your **blood volume** and **red blood cells** increase, your **heart rate** becomes faster, your **lungs** enlarge, taking in and absorbing more oxygen, your **muscles** expand and contract, your **energy** level increases, and your **nervous system** becomes less tense. The results of these activities will certainly give you a **stronger, trimmer figure.**

Your general appearance will be noticeably improved following your daily walk, since the walk will definitely improve your **digestion** and **circulation** and will enable you to ease away tension. Many people have noted a better night's **sleep** and disappearance of those **stress lines** around their eyes. Walking will also enable you to have better **posture** and a better **figure** following all of these changes that your body experiences by walking.

Your **complexion** will improve with walking, since there is nothing better for the complexion than the increased blood circulation to the skin. Medical research has even noted that **acne** problems improve,when walking is combined with medical treatment.

Muscle tone certainly is one of the most important results that you are looking for. After your daily walk, you will notice that your muscles will be toned and firm, and after you have been on your walking program for some time, you will notice that many of the fatty bulges and deposits on your body will decrease in size. Your **stomach** will flatten and your **calves** and **thighs** will become more trim, and your **buttocks muscles**

will become more proportioned. Many of these changes are due to improved muscle tone and, secondarily, to the strengthening of the spine.

Studies have shown that the circulatory system can increase the amount of oxygen to many parts of the body, even to the **hair.** Many of us who have lackluster, dry hair will notice an improvement in the appearance of the hair after a walking program. The hair, because of its increase in protein content, due to increased blood flow, will gain more life and it will become glossier and appear healthier.

Walking, therefore, is as **natural** as breathing and as helpful as an adequate night's sleep. Walking not only trims you down, but firms up your muscles. Walking is actually the only non-strenuous exercise that is relaxing, healthy, and beautifying, and can be part of a regular program of **health** and **beauty care.**

Remember, it is not necessary to kill yourself in order to stay fit and trim. Walking produces the same figure control and aerobic fitness benefits as does jogging and other strenuous exercises without the potential dangers. The fact remains that exercise does not have to be painful in order to be effective and beneficial.

THE MYTH OF CELLULITE

Cellulite is a different kind of fat requiring special types of treatment to get rid of it. **False!**

Fat is fat, and cellulite is actually a **myth.** When fat cells immediately beneath the skin enlarge, sometimes the strands of fibrous tissue that connect these fat cells don't stretch. This gives ordinary fat a lumpy appearance on the hips, thighs and buttocks, which has been given the mythical name – **cellulite**, by gimmick diet promoters.

In a recent study conducted at Johns Hopkins University in Baltimore, fat biopsies (small pieces of tissue) were taken from people with lumpy, fatty tissues (the mythical cellulite) and from people with regular fat deposits. The result: All of the biopsy specimens were identified under the microscope as **ordinary fat cells.** There was no tissue identified as cellulite!

Any product claiming to be a special treatment designed to get rid of "cellulite" is phony. The Food & Drug Administration has recently published a booklet entitled "Cellulite," in an effort to protect the public from spending money for a magical cure for a mythical disorder. Write to the Consumer Information Center, Dept. 560K, Pueblo, CO 81009 for a free copy of this booklet.

PHYSICAL EFFECTS OF A WALKING PROGRAM

The following physical and physiological effects will be noted after you have been on your walking diet for a six-week period:

1. **Flatter stomach** – the abdominal muscles will be firm and support the intra-abdominal contents, which give the appearance and the reality of a flatter stomach.
2. **Slender thighs** – leg strengthening and loss of fat in the thigh muscles will reduce the outer and inner thigh dimensions.
3. **Firmer buttocks** – the large buttocks muscle, called the gluteus maximus, will contract and draw the buttocks higher and make them appear firmer.
4. **Upper arms leaner and shapelier** – the muscles of the upper arm, which include the triceps and biceps, will increase their muscle tone, and the fat loss from the fleshy part of the upper arm will combine to form a firmer, shapelier arm.
5. **Firmer, higher appearing breasts** – the pectoral muscles of the chest will lift the breasts to make them appear larger and firmer.
6. **Increased level of energy** – with increased aerobic training, the lungs, heart, and circulation will be improved in efficiency and add more energy to your day.

7.   **Improved nightly sleep** – a regular walking program will aid in sleep without the use of sedatives or tranquilizers.

8.   **Improved cardio-vascular fitness**—your heart muscle will pump blood more efficiently which will help to lower your blood pressure and improve your over-all circulation.

9.   **Physical fitness and stamina**—will improve as you continue on your walking program.

10.   **Weight-loss and weight-maintenance**—walking burns calories, which burns fat which in turn results in weight-loss that stays lost forever.

TIP # 90
"NO PAIN – NO GAIN" – NOT TRUE!

Finally, recent medical research on heart disease is at last stating what I've been telling my patients and readers for the past twenty years: that moderate exercise prevents heart disease. I've always contended that exercise doesn't have to be stressful, painful, or exhausting in order for it to be beneficial. In my previous articles and books, I've refuted the exercise enthusiasts who followed the mantra **"no pain – no gain,"** with reference to fitness development. This theory is pure baloney! Strenuous, painful exercise regimes are no more effective than a moderate walking program at 3 mph, in order to develop cardiovascular fitness and good health. In fact, strenuous exercises are more likely to do more harm than good.

I've also stated over and over again to my patients and in my books that the so-called **"target heart-rate zone" is just a myth!** No one has ever proven scientifically that a rapid heart rate is essential for cardiovascular fitness. In fact, it could be extremely dangerous to keep the heart beating rapidly for long periods of time, especially in individuals who have undiagnosed preexisting heart disease. The most important proven fact is that strenuous exercise is not only hazardous, but it is counterproductive to cardiovascular fitness and good health. Strenuous, short bursts of anaerobic exercises contribute nothing towards the prevention of heart disease and strokes, and, in fact, strenuous exercise may actually cause a heart attack or a stroke! These potentially serious consequences may be the result of strenuous exercises raising the blood pressure to dangerous levels or by causing the heart to beat irregularly (cardiac arrhythmias).

In a recent study of over 17,000 women and men, it was concluded that *moderate exercise* is an independent factor in the prevention of deaths by cardiovascular diseases. The American Heart Association presented the following findings:

·   Despite blood pressure, cholesterol, or age, moderate exercise has an independent effect in preventing heart disease and strokes.

·   Men in the lower 20% of physical fitness had a 50% higher incidence for heart disease than men falling between the 30-50% range of fitness development.

·   Women in the bottom 20% zone of fitness, however, had a 70% higher incidence of heart disease than those women in the 30-50% range of fitness development.

·   The major conclusion was that "just a little bit of exercise" is all that is needed to lower your risk of cardiovascular disease. And I think it is a bit ironic that the report ended with my longstanding quotation: *"You don't need to run a marathon in order to reduce your risk of heart disease."*

Researchers at the Disease Control Center in Atlanta revealed a startling finding after reviewing 43 previous studies on heart disease. The one statistically significant, predisposing factor in the development of heart disease, which appeared in every single study, was a *lack of exercise*. Their research revealed that people who exercised the least had almost twice the risk of developing heart disease as those who exercised regularly. This particular study brought together the findings of the 43 previous studies, which had all measured physical activity in many different ways. Walking was as effective as any other type of exercise in preventing heart disease without the added risk of injury and disability, which occurred in the more strenuous exercises. This analysis suggests that the lack of exercise on its own may be as strong a risk factor for developing heart disease as high blood pressure, smoking, and high cholesterol. The Disease Control Center also stated that about 95% of adults in the USA get little or no exercise at all. *Don't sit around and get obese. Otherwise, you're at risk for heart disease!*

TIP # 91
WALKING WEIGHT-LOSS TIPS

How many times have you heard someone, or even perhaps yourself, say, *"I'm giving up. Exercise is boring."* Over 65% of people who start an exercise program abandon it after four to six weeks. Surprising, isn't it? Not really! Initial enthusiasm is often quickly replaced by boredom. Most of the exercise equipment and athletic clothes quickly find their way into the recesses of the closet.

Walking, fortunately, is one of the only exercises that the majority of people continue on a regular basis. The percentage of people who give up walking as a regular form of exercise is less than 25% of those who start on a walking program. Perhaps, it is because walking doesn't require special equipment or clothing. Or perhaps it's because there are no clubs to join or dues to pay. Or perhaps it's just that most walkers are usually rugged individualists and are more determined than most to keep in good shape. I think the real reason that walkers stay with their walking program is simply that *walking is fun!* And isn't that what an exercise should be? True, we all want physical fitness, good health, weight control, and longevity. But most of all we want an escape from the stress of everyday living. Walking provides a stress-free, fun-filled activity that we can do anyplace, anywhere, anytime. Here are some tips to keep your walking program interesting, enjoyable, and, most of all, filled with fun. And besides, you'll actually be losing weight without even realizing it.

1. ***Don't expect results too soon.*** Whether it's weight control or physical fitness that you're looking for, remember, "Rome wasn't built in a day and neither were you." Give you body time to adapt to your regular walking program.

2. ***Make your walking program convenient and flexible***. The more adaptable you are to when and where you walk, the more likely you are to do it on a regular basis.

3.   *Vary your walking program*. Vary your walking times (morning, afternoon or evening), depending on your schedule.

4.   *Change your walking route every week or two*. If near home or work, walk in a different direction and observe, feel, and smell new sights, sounds, and odors on your new route. The road less traveled may be the most fun.

5.   *Keep a record of your walking program*. For example, how long did you walk today, and approximately how far did you walk? Record the time and location of your walk and your impressions of the area in which you walked. Maybe it's an area you'd like to stay away from or one you'd like to explore again.

6.   *Record your weight only once every week* to see if you are losing the amount of weight you'd like to lose, or if you are just walking to maintain your present weight. Remember, walkers who want to maintain their present weight usually can have a bonus snack every day without gaining an ounce.

7.   *Either walk alone or with a friend or relative.* Walking can be a social activity, as well as an exercise. Spending time with someone you like or love can certainly add to the enjoyment of your walking program. Walking is one of the only exercises that lets you talk as you walk. If you are unable to talk because of shortness of breath, then you're probably walking too fast.

8.   *Take a walk-break instead of a coffee break.* Walking actually clears the mind and puts vitality and energy back into your body's walking machine. Coffee and a donut add caffeine and sugar to your body's sitting machine. Both the caffeine and sugar cause your insulin production to increase, because of the initial rise in blood sugar. This insulin surge then causes a sharp drop in your blood sugar. So instead of coming back to work invigorated as you

do from a walk-break, you come back fatigued, light-headed, and hungry from a coffee-donut-break.

9. ***Walk a dog or a pedometer.*** Studies show that dog owners, who actually walk their dogs, have a built-in incentive to stay on a walking program. If you're not a dog person, but need a hook to hang your walking program on, there are a number of shops that sell pedometers to keep track of the miles that you walk. Many stores also carry walking sticks for dress or protection when you walk. These sticks can also help you climb hills if you are hiking and can act as a handy weapon if you have need to use one.

10. ***Don't be afraid to take a break for a few days or even a week.*** Any exercise program, even one as easy and fun-filled as walking, can eventually become a little tiring. A few days' break from your schedule will give you a short breather so that you can return to your walking program with renewed interest and enthusiasm. Remember, you won't gain all of your weight back or get out of shape if you take an occasional break from your walking program.

11. ***Never exercise if you are injured or ill.*** Your body needs time to heal and recuperate from whatever ails you. Remember, you can't exercise through an injury or an illness. Many so-called fitness nuts have tried this with disastrous results. For example, a strained muscle has been aggravated into a fractured bone or a simple cold has turned into pneumonia. Listen to your body. It's smarter than your brain.

12. ***Promise yourself a treat when you stick to your walking program.*** For example – a bouquet of flowers, a night at the theatre, a movie, a ball game, a new dress, or a weekend away. Indulge yourself. You deserve it!

13. ***Get a complete physical from your physician.*** Before starting any exercise plan, even one as moderate as walking, you should consult your own physician for a complete physical examination.

TIP # 92
INDOOR DIET-STEP® TIPS

Don't wait until the "weather is better" to go out and walk. There's no excuse for not exercising at home on any day when the weather is too cold or windy. Also, take precautions against exercising when it's very hot or humid outdoors. Heat exhaustion and, occasionally, heat stroke are complications frequently found in those crazy jogging nuts that you see running on hot, humid days. Remember, it's not necessary to walk outdoors if the weather is extremely cold, windy, wet, hot, or humid.

1.   STATIONARY DIET-STEP®:
This is a combination of walking and running in place. Walk in place for 5 minutes, lifting your foot approximately 4 inches off the floor and taking approximately 60 steps a minute (count only when right foot hits floor). Alternate this with 5 minutes of running in place, lifting your foot approximately 8 inches off the floor and taking approximately 90 steps a minute (again, only count when the right foot hits the floor). Use a padded exercise mat or a thick rug. Wear a padded sneaker or walking shoe. Bare feet will cause foot and leg injuries. Repeat this walk-run cycle (10 minutes total) two times daily for a total of 20 minutes. If you tire easily, stop and rest. I would rate this exercise – *Boring!*

2.   SKIPPING DIET-STEP®:
If you're coordinated enough to use a jump rope, skipping can be a fun indoor exercise. Skip over the rope, alternating one foot at a time for 5 minutes, and then skip using both feet together for 5 minutes. Use a mat or padded rug with a padded low sneaker or walking shoe. This 10-minute session can be repeated two times daily for a total of 20 minutes. If you feel you are not coordinated enough for rope skipping, then *skip it!*

3.   DANCE DIET-STEP®:
Turn on the music and dance to your favorite music, whether it's pop, jazz, classical, R&B, or any music with a moderately fast beat. Make

up your own moves and dance to the beat of the music. If you can keep it up for 20 minutes, good for you. Otherwise, two 10-minute sessions, separated by a rest period will still keep you aerobically fit.

4.   **STATIONARY BIKE DIET-STEP®:**
One of the easiest ways to continue your indoor weight-loss program is by using a stationary exercise bicycle. This is the only one-time investment you'll ever need to make as you travel the road towards fitness and good health. No other type of exercise equipment is necessary for your weight-loss program.

The most important features to look for in a stationary bicycle are a comfortable seat with good support, adjustable handlebars, a chain guard, a quiet pedal and chain, and a solid front wheel. Most come with speedometers to tell the rate that you are pedaling and odometers to tell the mileage that you pedal. An inexpensive stationary bike works just as well as an expensive one. Stationary bikes with moving handlebars are worthless. They claim to exercise the upper half of your body. In reality, they move your arms and back muscles passively, which can result in pulled muscles and strained ligaments.

The stationary bike is the safest and most efficient type of indoor exercise equipment that can be used in place of your outdoor walking program. You can listen to music, watch TV, talk on the telephone, or even read (a bookstand attachment can easily be clamped onto the handle bars) while riding your stationary bike. If the bike comes with a tension dial, leave it on zero or minimal tension. Remember, it is not necessary to strain yourself to develop aerobic fitness. Exercises like walking and the stationary bike can be fun, without being painful or stressful. You may alternate days of outdoor walking and indoor cycling, depending on your individual schedule.

You should pedal at a comfortable rate of between 10-15 miles/hour. To complete your daily exercise requirements, pedal for 20 minutes every day (divide into two 10-minute sessions to avoid fatigue). Always wear a walking shoe or sneaker (never pedal barefoot). A chain guard prevents clothing from getting caught in the bike chain; otherwise, roll up your sweats.

5.   TREADMILLS:
The treadmill is an effective way to burn calories and build cardiovascular fitness. Manual treadmills are hard on the feet, since you have to push down to make them move and the walking motion is unnatural. Look for motorized treadmills with a deck area (the walking space) with enough length and width to accommodate any stride. The deck area should be at least 18 inches wide by 55 inches long. A cushioned deck is better for your ankles and knees, and a thick tread belt is best. You can compare the thickness by the feel when you try out the treadmill, or by asking the salesman for the thickness measurement.

Look for motorized treadmills with a high continuous duty rating of at least 1.5 horsepower, as opposed to a motor with maximum output. Continuous duty motors give you constant maximum power, whereas maximum output motors surge to accommodate short spurts, but you won't be able to walk smoothly for an extended period of time. You can also choose a treadmill with a power incline; however, too much of an incline is bad for the knees and ankles and can put a strain on your back. Also, make sure that the machine has an automatic stop button, so, if you stumble or feel dizzy, you can push the button and halt the machine instantly.

6.   SWIMMING:
20 minutes of swimming provides the same aerobic conditioning and cardiovascular fitness benefits as walking and other indoor Diet-Step® exercises. Swimming, in fact, has the added benefit of being easy on the joints, especially if you have any form of arthritis or back problems. The reason for this is that swimming puts very little stress on the joints because of the decreased gravity factor provided by the buoyancy of the water. If you have access to an indoor or outdoor swimming pool, then 20 minutes of swimming will fit the bill perfectly for a weight-loss plan.

7.   ELLIPTICAL FITNESS MACHINES:
This type of machine combines the movement of a treadmill and a stair climber. Your feet loop forward to simulate walking, but the foot-

pads rise and fall with your feet. The elliptical motion provides a no-impact type of exercise, which is great if you have arthritis or knee or back problems that make walking difficult. For maximum exercise, an elliptical machine with dual cross-trainer arms, which move back and forth as you stride, rather than the stationary arms, provides maximum exercise and burns more calories, and uses more muscle groups.

Most of these machines come with an adjustable ramp incline and resistance settings. However, the normal setting is usually more than adequate for cardiovascular fitness. Also, be careful of small space-saving elliptical machines, since they may not comfortably accommodate a tall person's stride or may not afford full range of motion. Many people, however, complain that the elliptical motion feels unnatural, not at all like walking. They feel as if you have to pull your feet up and then push them down to sustain the motion. Try out different machines to see if you're comfortable with this type of motion. If the motion feels awkward, unnatural, or strenuous, forget it.

8.   MALL WALKING:

For those of you who don't like to exercise at home when the weather's bad, an indoor mall can be just the place to take your 20-minute walk. Many malls open early before the stores open to accommodate "mall walkers." If you have access to one of these enclosed malls and don't like to stay at home exercising, then by all means get out there and do the Diet-Step®. Remember to put vigor, vim, and pep into your mall walk step. Keep your eyes straight ahead, so that you won't be window-shopping instead.

Caution: If any of these Diet-Step® indoor exercises cause excessive fatigue, weakness, shortness of breath, dizziness, headaches, chest pain, pain anywhere in the body, or any other unusual symptoms or signs, stop immediately and consult your physician.

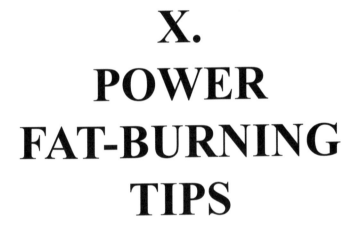

X.
POWER
FAT-BURNING
TIPS

TIP # 93
DROP IN, NOT OUT!

Why are there so many exercise dropouts? And why don't many people even try to begin an exercise plan in the first place? Most individuals in these categories think that an exercise program is futile, since they'll never be able to look like the perfect bodies in the magazines or at the gym. They actually give up before they even start exercising, because of being intimidated.

Most people think physical fitness is actually harder than it is. And they feel that exercise programs are too complicated, when they hear terms like "oxygen consumption," "body fat composition," body mass index," "lean muscle mass," etc. It all sounds too complicated and too boring for most of us to begin exercising in any formalized program.

What many people don't realize is that you don't have to participate in a regimented exercise program to see results. They don't have to join a gym or health club and be intimidated by a 24-year-old fitness instructor with boundless energy. And they don't have to exercise vigorously or do strenuous exercises in order to obtain maximum fitness and a lean, trim body. As we've already discussed, exercise doesn't have to be strenuous to see results. Exercise doesn't have to be painful in order to be gainful. You don't have to be put into a situation where you feel intimidated by an instructor in a gym or on a video-tape.

Exercise can really be fun! It can be easy to follow and easy to continue. It doesn't have to be boring or a drudgery that has to be done. That's why the 20-Minute Diet-Step® Plan was devised – in order to make it easy for people to become fit and trim, and to make it easy for them to maintain their new levels of fitness. Remember the two exercise myths we've discussed in Tip # 90 – ("No Pain – No Gain" and the "Target Heart Rate Zone"). Both of these so-called exercise precepts are what makes many people discontinue their exercise plans or never start them in the first place. Once you realize that it is not necessary to make exercise painful or stressful, you can begin to relax and enjoy the Diet-Step® Walking Plan.

IT TAKES LONGER TO GET OUT OF SHAPE
THAN IT DOES TO GET INTO SHAPE

What if I can't keep up with the exercise plan regularly? What if I have to stop for a few days or a week, or even longer, if some interruption in my life prevents me from continuing? This is the kind of thinking that prevents many people from starting an exercise program and prevents others from going back to one that they've already begun. Never fear, the answer's here – *"It takes much longer to get out of shape than it does to get into shape."*

The Diet-Step® Plan is forgiving. Even if you miss a few days or a week, or a few weeks in a month, there is no need to worry. Once you have been conditioned physically, it takes a lot longer to get out of shape than it took you to get into shape. The rate of regression depends on how long you've been exercising and how fit you are. The body is remarkable, since it tends to hold onto these fitness gains long after you've stopped exercising. Most people lose muscle strength at about one-half the rate at which they gained it. So, if you've been doing the Diet-Step® Plan for three months and have to discontinue for any reason, it could take up to six months for your body to fall back to its pre-training state.

If you've been walking for approximately 2-3 months your aerobic capacity starts to decrease in the first two to three weeks after you've stopped exercising, but it can take almost six to eight months before fit exercisers get back to the pre-fitness level where they started. Aerobic exercising (walking) decreases the LDL (bad cholesterol) and increases the HDL (good cholesterol) after you've been on your walking program for approximately two to three months. Studies show that it took at least three months for those cholesterol levels to return to their original pre-walking workout levels after the exercise of walking was discontinued. That's pretty good, considering you've stopped walking all that time. When walkers resumed their walking program, it took them only one-half the time to return to their original levels of fitness.

So, don't worry if you have to discontinue your walking program for any reason or for any period of time. The benefits that you've worked so hard for are long lasting and they are easily obtained again in one-half the time. *The Diet-Step® Plan is forgiving and it keeps on giving!*

WHAT'S THE BEST TIME TO DO THE DIET-STEP®

You can do your 20-minute Diet-Step Walking Plan any time of the day that's convenient for you. It's your schedule, so make it any time that you'd like. You can also change the times that you exercise each day depending on your own individual work schedule or home activities. Here are the pros and cons of exercising at various times of the day according to the so-called fitness experts. Take it with a grain of salt and individualize your own schedule to your own liking.

Morning – The main obstacle in the morning is getting out of bed. Once you're up, depending on if you're an early riser or not, you may want to leave yourself enough time so that you won't be rushed, especially if you have to go to work or have home responsibilities. Since there are usually few disruptions in the A.M., many people who walk in the morning are more likely to stick with their exercise plans over a long period of time. Plus, the sense of accomplishment, having completed your exercise early in the day, gives you a psychological rush for the first part of the day.

Afternoon – Most individuals feel an energy lag between 2:00 and 3:00 in the afternoon, which is related to the body's natural circadian rhythm. It may also be partly due to having just eaten lunch. Some exercise physiologists say that walking midday can smooth out that energy lag by increasing the levels of certain hormones that will perk you up for several hours. Remember, however, that it is not a good idea to exercise immediately after lunch or to skip lunch altogether. Walking for

20 minutes and then eating a light lunch will boost your energy level for the rest of the day.

Evening – Due to fluctuations in biological rhythms, it is in the late afternoon or early evening when your breathing is easier because your lungs' airways open wider, your muscle strength increases due to a slightly higher body temperature, and your joints and muscles are at their most flexible. This may also be a good time to walk according to some exercise physiologists. However, if you've had an extremely difficult day, and if you're dead tired, then revving yourself up for exercise may seem more like a chore than fun. Also, never exercise near bedtime, since the increased energy levels that follow the exercise may make it difficult to fall asleep.

Remember, however, that the choice is yours. Do the Diet-Step® according to your own biological clock and how you feel, and also according to your own time schedule. It's your body, so listen to it, and it will respond to you with boundless energy and pep when you do the Diet-Step®.

TIP # 94
HOW TO OVERCOME DIET PLATEAU

There invariably comes a point when after you've dieted and lost weight, that you reach a plateau, where you can't lose any more weight, no matter how hard you try. No matter how many calories you reduce from your diet, your weight doesn't budge. You're actually stuck in diet plateau land, which can be very disheartening and often leads you to abandon your diet efforts. The only way to break through this plateau is to increase your aerobic exercise and beef-up your strength-training activity. Aerobic activities such as walking, jumping rope, dancing, tennis and other sports including indoor exercises like the treadmill, will increase your calorie-burning aerobic fitness activity. Aerobic exercise burns extra calories that you can't possibly lose by dieting alone. Walking for 20 minutes a day can improve your cardio-vascular fitness while you burn unwanted fat calories, which helps you break the diet plateau. In 4-6 weeks time, you'll see those extra stubborn pounds melt away as you successfully reach your target weight.

With the addition of strength-training exercises to your aerobic activity, you will begin to build muscle mass, which increases your body's metabolic rate. This means that the additional lean muscle mass that you develop during weight-training will help you burn calories at a faster rate, even when you're at rest. One pound of lean muscle burns ten times as many calories as a pound of fat. Weight-training, therefore, is the added boost that helps you to break through that stubborn weight plateau. So the real secret to beating the diet plateau is to follow a healthy diet, to engage in an aerobic fat-burning activity like walking and to build lean muscle mass with easy strength-training exercises. The combination of these three components will reshape your body as you lose those difficult unwanted pounds.

WALK IT OFF!

The biggest diet fallacy is that people think they're overweight because they eat too many calories. That's only one-half of the problem. The second half of the problem is that people don't really get enough exercise to burn these calories off.

If you really want to lose weight and keep the weight off permanently, then you have to start exercising regularly. And there is no better exercise than a regular walking program. If you walk regularly, you'll not only lose those unwanted pounds, but you've discovered the secret of keeping the weight off permanently. Weight-loss, which is secondary to an aerobic exercise like walking, becomes permanently lost.

Interestingly enough, you get the same weight-loss and fitness benefits by walking every day as you would from joining a gym. People who walk regularly every day for 20 minutes had the same fat-burning, weight-loss benefits, fitness improvement, and regulation of blood pressure as did people who worked out vigorously at a gym four to five days per week.

The added bonus of a regular walking program is that you actually continue to burn calories after you stop walking. You will continue to burn fat, which essentially burns calories, for many hours after your aerobic walking exercise program is finished.

This continued fat-burning effect is due to the increase in basal metabolic rate that occurs after you've walked. This calorie-burning process can continue even while you are resting or sleeping due to the increase in your metabolic rate that was primed during your daily walking program.

It actually takes time for the metabolic rate to slow down after exercise, which is why you can eat extra calories after walking without actually gaining any weight. And before your body has a chance to slow down its metabolic rate, you will be walking again, either later the same day or the next day. Your body starts to get used to this higher basal metabolic rate, and therefore runs at a higher speed daily. The result: More calories burned per day, which results in increased weight-loss and a decrease in rebound weight gained. In other words, weight that continues to be lost is essentially lost forever.

The opposite is also true. Little or no exercise translates into a slower metabolic rate. This means you'll burn fewer calories than you take in and weight gain gradually ensues. Excess calories go straight to your storage fat cells where they comfortably rest. The result, of course, is excess fat storage in your abdomen, buttocks, hips, and thighs.

Physical activity like an aerobic walking program actually cuts your appetite by suppressing the brain's appetite control center. The brain reasons that if you are exercising, then you shouldn't be eating. This results in less hunger, less calories consumed, and thus less weight gain. As you burn extra calories, you will also boost your energy level. This extra energy will produce a feeling of well-being and will help you to want to continue with your aerobic exercise-walking program on a regular basis. You will not only be happy and motivated, but you will get thin in the process. Aerobics lead to a boost in energy and increase endorphins, which result in a feeling of well-being. Now you will be thin, happy, motivated, and energetic.

PUMP UP MUSCLES AND BURN FAT

Studies reported at the 2004 Experimental Biology Meeting in Washington showed that short, simple, weight-training workouts helped men and women lose weight and keep that weight off permanently. Weight-training also was shown to strengthen the body's immune system, as well as lower the blood pressure.

By following a low-fat, moderate protein and complex carbohydrate diet, combined with simple weight-training exercises for fourteen weeks, the participants in this study lost fat and weight, and increased the proportion of muscle to body weight. Also, these men and women showed significant improvements in blood pressure, heart rate, and aerobic fitness.

Another similar study showed that middle-aged and elderly people developed stronger muscles and a healthier immune system while walking regularly, combined with light weight-training exercises. Many of the middle-aged and elderly people in this study were moderately obese when they started the program. After twelve weeks, the majority of the obese participants had lost considerable weight, in addition to gaining lean muscle mass. These individuals also developed improved cardiovascular fitness, in addition to gaining muscle strength and boosting their energy levels.

TIP # 95
POWER-DIET-STEP®

A FIGURE SUPREME— A BODY THAT'S LEAN

Strength training is essential for weight control, muscle strengthening, skeletal health, and overall well-being in both women and men. Aerobic exercise is great for cardiovascular health and burning calories, but it does not necessarily build upper body muscle strength. Fat replaces muscles as people age, unless they exercise to offset this natural process. The necessity for strength training is even more pronounced in women because they begin with more fat cells and less muscle tissue compared with men.

Women and men after the age of 35 lose muscle mass at a rate of approximately one-third to one-half pound per year. Strength training exercises, using lightweight, handheld weights while walking, make muscles stronger and strengthen the skeleton. The bones strengthen because the weights cause the muscles to contract. These muscles and ligaments then create a traction or tension on the bone, thus causing the bone to strengthen by absorbing more calcium from the bloodstream and losing less calcium from the bone. This process increases the mineral content of the bones, thus strengthening the bones and making them less brittle as you age.

Many studies have shown that people who engage in strength training exercises develop an increased skeletal muscle mass of approximately 1.5 kilograms, whereas sedentary people lose 0.5-kilogram muscle mass over a one-year period. Likewise, bone mineral density increased by 1% in the strength training group, and decreased by 2.5% in the sedentary group. Also, these studies showed that strength training in men and women increased their lean muscle mass by 4% and decreased their fat mass by 8%.

What do all these numbers mean? They mean that your muscles will become more defined and shapely and you will feel stronger because your muscles are actually stronger. You will have better balance and greater joint flexibility. You will feel more energetic and more confident. Your bones will be structurally stronger and less likely to break as you get older.

You will be less likely to develop osteoporosis or thinning of the bones as you get older. In other words, you will have *"a body that's lean and a figure supreme."*

STRENGTH TRAINING

Weight resistance exercises are not only good for your muscles, but are also good for the body's most important muscle – the heart. In a recent report released by the American Heart Association, there is now increasing evidence that strength training can favorably modify many risk factors for heart disease, including blood cholesterol and triglycerides, blood pressure, body fat levels, and glucose metabolism. Until recently, the conventional thinking was that strength training exercises helped to build and sculpt your muscles, but did little to help the cardiovascular system and, in fact, might even be harmful to your heart. This current study released by the American Heart Association dispels many of the myths and misconceptions regarding strength training. The current study showed that strength training is not in the least harmful if one is reasonable and not trying to be a power weightlifter.

In addition to this special report by the American Heart Association, which was published in the Journal of Circulation in February 2000, another related study was also released in February 2000 in the Journal of Hypertension. This study showed that weight strength training exercises could significantly lower blood pressure. Those women who regularly lifted light weights experienced a reduction in resting systolic blood pressure (when your heart muscles contract) and a reduction in the resting diastolic blood pressure (when your heart muscles relax). Their resting blood pressures dropped regardless of their body composition, whether they performed heavy weight resistance exercises with longer rest periods or lighter weight exercises with shorter rest periods.

POWER DIET-STEP®

The Power Diet-Step® plan is simply a combination of walking for 20 minutes with hand-held weights. This combines the aerobic benefits of walking with the strength-training benefits of lifting light weights. You will be walking with 1 or 2 pound hand-held weights in each hand. They come either with a strap that goes around the back of your hand or they are fitted with grooves that you grip your fingers into. So you will see that the Power Diet-Step® Walking Workout Plan will not only make you feel and look great, but helps to strengthen your heart and lower your blood pressure. In addition, it sculpts and molds your body into a figure supreme and a body that's lean. Not a bad combination for a 20-minute walking workout 2 or 3 times a week. In any event, everyone should have a complete physical examination before using handheld light-weights while walking.

BOOST ENERGY

For people who have reached a plateau in weight-loss, the ideal fat burner is pumping up your walking workouts with handheld weights. I usually recommend 1-pound cushioned handheld weights, with either straps attached that encircle the palms of your hands or with padded grooves for your fingers to grip. After using the 1-pound weights with walking for about 4-6 weeks, I advise my patients to graduate to the 2-pound weights. These weights should be cushioned and covered with rubber or vinyl, since they don't rust and aren't cold to use in cold weather. If the 2-pound weights seem too heavy, then stay with the 1-pound weights.

Walkers burn approximately 25% more calories doing the Power Diet-Step® using handheld weights. Also, walking with weights builds lean muscle mass, which burns an additional 50 calories an hour per 1 pound of muscle. This activity is excellent for people of all ages and helps to maintain strong rotator cuff and shoulder muscles. Walking with weights also helps to develop good muscle tone, which improves balance and stability when walking. Also, walking with handheld weights helps you to develop good posture and strong chest and abdominal wall muscles.

The Power Diet-Step® is the ideal combination of an aerobic exercise, which also combines upper body strength training. There is no need to engage in strenuous aerobic exercises or to lift heavy weights at the gym (either free weights or machine weights) to achieve cardiovascular fitness, weight-loss, and improved lean muscle mass. Your body will burn fat as you lose weight and you will develop a new and improved, lean and firm figure. This results from the aerobic fat-burning exercise of walking and the strength-training, muscle development of walking with hand-held weights.

These changes occur because of the combination of the fat-burning aerobic walking exercise and the strength-training, muscle-building exercise when you use handheld weights while walking. This is a combination that is truly impossible to reproduce. You don't have to do separate aerobic and strength-training exercises at different times or on different days. It's all combined in one easy, user-friendly exercise. Walking with weights just 2-3 days per week is all that you'll need to develop cardiovascular fitness, permanent weight-loss, and a trim, firm figure. Both men and women benefit from the Power Diet-Step®. This exercise is ideal in helping to prevent osteoporosis, since walking with handheld weights puts the necessary tension on the bones and muscles, which is essential in preventing bone loss. The Power Diet-Step® plan of walking with weights is essential in helping to improve cardiovascular fitness, thus lowering blood pressure and also helping to reduce the incidence of heart disease and stroke.

The American Heart Association's finding in their latest study showed that weight resistance exercises should be of moderate intensity. In other words, instead of the fallacy "no pain, no gain," the truth, as I've always stated, is "train, don't strain."

TIP # 96
FIT, FIRM, FABULOUS YOU!

1.   Work Out While You Walk

No matter how hard or long you walk, your upper body, particularly your arms, gets a free ride. Upper body strength is only a small part of the walking motion. Even if you pump your arms vigorously, the essential problem remains, which is that your arms don't get stronger, since there is no resistance to encounter while you walk. Your legs encounter the resistance of the ground and support your body's weight when you're walking. In other words, your legs get stronger, your thighs, buttocks, and hips get firmer, and your abdomen gets flatter on just a walking program.

Weight resistance with handheld weights while walking, however, is a great way to put your arms to work and, at the same time, makes you a stronger walker. A walker's upper body should be geared towards strength and endurance, not building muscle bulk. In other words, we want to sculpt and mold the upper body (arms, back, and chest). The key to the Power Diet-Step® Walking Workout Plan is using light handheld weights while walking, which provides strength training.

2.   How Can Strength Training Exercises Help You Lose Weight?

When you walk with light handheld weights, you build muscle mass, which in turn speeds up your metabolism. Muscle tissue burns more calories than fat cells burn. Therefore, building muscle helps to boost your resting metabolism. This increase in the resting metabolism occurs because of the actual increased muscle mass that you develop and the increased metabolic activity in the muscles themselves. When combining your 20-minute aerobic walk with strength training exercises, you have the advantage of a "double blast" of calorie burning for weight-loss while trimming and toning your body. First of all, your aerobic walking burns approximately 360 calories per hour or 120 calories every 20 minutes. The strength training exercises using hand-held weights, burn another 360 calories per hour or 120 calories every 20 minutes, which is accomplished just by increasing the body's basal metabolism. Therefore, you are burning a total of 240 calories of fat every 20 minutes on the Power Diet-Step® Plan. So you can see you actually lose more weight, more quickly, by walking with handheld weights.

3.   Won't Weight Training Make Women's Muscles Bulky?

Women are afraid to train like men for fear of developing massive muscles. In reality, women don't have to fear turning into Arnold Schwarzenneger because of the increase in basal metabolic rate which occurs during the Power Diet-Step® Strength Training exercises. Remember, this is not power weight-lifting, this is a walking workout with handheld weights.

Since women have more body fat than men, they are less likely to bulk up like men, who have more muscle mass to begin with. Both men and women will see improvement in muscle tone and strength after only four to six weeks on the Power Diet-Step® Walking Workout. Muscles will become more defined and sculptured for a trim, firm look.

4.   How Often Should You Walk With Weights?

Studies show that strength-training exercises 2-3 times per week (not on consecutive days) prevent damage to your muscle fibers that need time to regenerate (heal) after being stressed with weight resistance exercises. Also, varying the muscle groups during strength training exercises helps to provide strength benefits to all of the upper body's muscles on a graduated basis. The beauty of the Power Diet-Step® Strength Training exercises is that they are done while you are walking, using very light weights. This decreases the possibility of muscle and ligament injury and eliminates the need for time-consuming regimented weightlifting routines. Newer research in exercise physiology has shown that working out a particular muscle group only twice a week offers the same strength and muscle toning benefits as working these muscles three times per week. What does this all mean? Well, on your Diet-Step® Walking Plan, you will be walking six days per week. It will only be necessary to use handheld weights on two days each week on your walking workout (Power Diet-Step®). If you desire more muscle toning and upper body strengthening exercises, you can increase the walking workout with handheld weights to three times per week.

5.   How Many Repetitions Should You Do With Each Exercise?

As you'll see from the following six Power Diet-Step® Walking Workout Exercises, it is only necessary to use handheld weights two days per week. You'll be able to customize the number of repetitions for each exercise depending on your own comfort level. Doing one set of 10-12 repetitions for each exercise is usually adequate as you rotate from one exercise to another during your 20-minute walk. You can do more repetitions later on in your training program, if your muscles don't become sore or if you don't tire easily. Remember to start slowly with fewer repetitions when you start your walking workout and gradually build up the number of repetitions until you reach your own comfort level. You will however, be using the natural arm swing motion (see walking workout exercise #1) most of the time during your 20-minute walk.

****

The Power Diet-Step® Walking Workout Plan makes your body leaner and your muscles more defined and sculptured. In addition, this plan builds stronger bones and muscles, straightens your posture, and strengthens your joints and ligaments. This plan also boosts your metabolism, which, in turn, helps you to lose weight. And finally, strength training exercises using the hand-held weights, enhances your sense of well-being and your self-confidence. In other words, a new, vital, improved you will be full of pep when you do the Power Diet-Step®.

TIP # 97
WALKING WORKOUTS

1.   Natural Arm Swing Power Diet-Step®

This is the most common arm motion that you use when walking. Place your arms hand down naturally at your side, holding weights with palms facing your body. As you walk, alternately swing your arms gently, as you bend your elbows slightly. This is the natural arm motion of walking that you use during your regular six-day-per-week Diet-Step® walking weight-loss plan. This exercise strengthens your triceps and upper shoulder muscles. This is the natural arm swing motion that you'll be using most of the time during your 20-minute walk. Keep your arms swinging naturally, so that the weights do not create a dead load on your joints.

2.   Locomotive Arm Motion Power Diet-Step®

This is the arm motion that you see joggers use while they are running. Hold your arms bent at approximately 90° at the elbow. Hold weights with palms facing your body. Now, do the locomotive! Alternately, move your arms forward and backward. You will feel the muscles of your upper arm, triceps, and shoulder strengthen as you do the locomotive.

3.   Hammer Curl Power Diet-Step®

This exercise starts out like exercise No. 1 (natural arm swing), arms at your sides, holding weights with palms facing body. As you walk, bend each arm alternately at the elbow toward your shoulder, and then lower arm to the side of your leg. Pretend you're hammering a nail into a tabletop. This exercise strengthens your forearm and biceps muscles.

This exercise is safer to do while walking than is the traditional biceps curl, where your palms face away from your body. You prevent the handheld weights from bumping your legs as you walk when you do the hammer curl instead of the traditional biceps curl. Also, you get better muscle strengthening and toning with this exercise.

4.   **Flap Your Wings Power Diet-Step®**

Hold weights next to the sides of your legs, palms facing in. Lift both arms together, out to your sides and away from your body. Lift arms out to the level of your shoulders (no higher) as you walk, and then lower both arms to your sides. This exercise must be done carefully while you're walking; otherwise, you may lose your balance or bump into someone who is abreast of you while you walk. If you find that this exercise is too difficult to do while walking, then wait until your walk is finished and then do 10-12 repetitions of the Flap Your Wings Power Diet-Step®. This exercise strengthens your upper back, chest, and shoulder muscles.

5.   **Reach For The Sky Power Diet-Step®**

Think of this exercise as lifting the world off your shoulders as you reach for the sky. Hold arms out to sides, elbows bent in line with chest. Hold weights in arms, palms facing forward at shoulder level. Now, reach for the sky! Raise weights above head, until arms are fully extended. Then lower weights back down to shoulder level. This exercise sculpts and strengthens the upper back and shoulder muscles.

6.   **Butterfly Power Diet-Step®**

Hold weights in each hand in front of you at chest level, palms facing each other and elbows bent at 90°. Raise both arms out to your sides like a butterfly. Then bring weights back together in front of you at chest level. Be careful not to bang your hands together. This exercise is particularly good for developing and sculpting mid-chest and upper back muscles.

If you find this exercise is too difficult to do while walking, then you can do it at the end of your 20-minute walk. If you're tired, you can even do this exercise lying down, as follows:

a.   Lie on your back, with knees bent and feet on the floor.

b.   Start with arms stretched out above you, towards the ceiling, with weights in each hand, with palms facing each other.

c.   Slowly lower your arms out to the sides, and then pull arms back to starting position. Use primarily your chest muscles while doing this exercise, not your arm muscles.

WALKING WORKOUT EXERCISE TIPS

1.   Start with 1-pound hand-held weights for the first 4-6 weeks, and then build up to 2-pound weights after you feel comfortable walking with your 1-pound hand-held weights. If you find that 2-pound weights are too heavy, then stick with the 1-pound weights. You'll still get the same great muscle strengthening, toning, and sculpting benefits.

2.   Tighten your abdominal muscles while you are doing these walking workout exercises. This will help to provide support for your upper body while toning and flattening your abdominal muscles.

3.   Don't overdo or over stretch while doing any of these exercises, since the risk of muscle and tendon injury increases as the weights are swung in greater arcs. If any particular exercise feels uncomfortable, then stop it immediately.

4.   You can vary the exercises as you walk. Remember to stop any particular exercise if you become tired or your muscles become sore. If you find that any of the exercises are too difficult to do while you walk (particularly exercises # 4, 5, or 6), then do them at the end of your walk. Only do 10-12 repetitions of each exercise while you are standing still.

5.   The six Power Diet-Step exercises only have to be done 2 or 3 days per week (not on consecutive days), to achieve maximum strength-training and muscle toning benefits. If the weather is bad, then you can do 10-12 repetitions of each exercise at home after you complete your 20-minute indoor exercise workout (see Tip # 92).

6.   Let's say it's a hot day or any day that you don't want to use your hand-held weights. You can carry a 16 or 20 ounce plastic bottle of water in each hand during your 20-minute walk. You can do your Power Diet-Step exercises with the water bottles. As you walk, you can drink alternately from each bottle as you gradually lighten your load. When you're finished, you'll feel refreshed and re-hydrated.

TIP # 98
POWER STRETCH

Stretching exercises can improve the flexibility of the joints, muscles, and tendons, thus making the body less prone to injury. Stretching also increases the flow of blood to the stretched muscle and helps to promote bone growth where there is a stretching motion against gravity. There is increasing evidence that stretching has a calming effect on the central nervous system by transmitting relaxing signals along chemical neurotransmitter pathways from the peripheral nervous system to the brain.

Stretching should be done slowly, and stretching one muscle group at a time is preferable. For instance, stretch both arms in front of you and hold that position for 30 seconds, and then let your arms down slowly, and relax them for an additional 30 seconds. Repeat this extension of both arms out to your sides, holding for 30 seconds, and then slowly letting them down and relaxing them for 30 seconds. Repeat this motion with your arms above your head, and then with your hands clasped in back of your head with your elbows bent, as if you are stretching when you get out of bed.

During each of these exercises, gently stretch the arms by actually pulling or pushing them away from the body, and then pulling them back towards the body. Remember to do it gently, and if it hurts, you're stretching your muscles too much. Do the same procedure with your neck muscles. First look up and hold your head in that position for 30 seconds and then relax, returning to a normal head position for 30 seconds. Repeat the same procedure looking to the left, and then to the right. Also, repeat this looking down, with your chin resting on your chest for 30 seconds, and then return to the normal position for 30 seconds.

The best way to stretch your leg muscles and ligaments is to sit in a chair and stretch one leg at a time in front of you for 30 seconds, then relax the muscles, and then bend your knee and hold that position for an additional 30 seconds, then relax the muscles and place your foot back on the floor. Repeat the same procedure with the other leg. You also can accomplish the same thing by pressing your feet into a footrest while sitting on a plane, train, bus, or at your desk.

These simple stretching exercises are designed to develop maximum flexibility of the muscles, ligaments, and joints. Although not as elaborate as yoga or tai chi, they are effective limbering and toning exercises for the body. These stretching steps help prepare the body for mental as well as physical fitness. These exercises help you to get in touch with your body as you contemplate the slow, relaxing stretching steps. Remember also to take slow, deep breaths during the stretching exercises for maximum relaxing techniques.

You can develop any stretching routine that feels good to you, not just those described above. Stretching is an individual exercise, and what feels good for one person may not be satisfactory to another person. Stretching can be done also by interlacing the fingers in front of your body, above your head, or behind your back.

Remember, if the stretching exercise hurts, either during or after the exercise, then you have stretched too vigorously. Go easy the next time. When you've finished, your muscles should feel relaxed, not taut or tight. The major advantage of the Power Stretch is that it can be done any time, anywhere, or anyplace. When you don't have the time to walk or the weather's inclement, stretching is a viable alternative to limbering up. Stretching can also be used in conjunction with the Diet- Step Walking Plan or the Power Diet-Step Walking Workouts for a leaner, trimmer figure. Power stretching before your workout has the advantages of getting your muscles and ligaments tuned and toned up before your walk with or without weights. Stretching also has the advantage of preventing muscle and ligament injuries when you walk or work out.

TIP # 99
STAY STRONG & LOOK GREAT!

One of the easiest and most effective ways to fight bone loss is to walk regularly every day. Walking puts the necessary tension on the ligaments and tendons, which are attached to your bones, while keeping them strong and preventing calcium loss from the bones. Bones that do not have this chronic tension-type pull from ligaments and tendons start to gradually leak calcium into the bloodstream. By walking every day, you keep your bones strong by preventing the loss of calcium from the bones.

If you don't exercise enough, then you are particularly subject to developing osteoporosis, especially if you are a woman over the age of 50. Osteoporosis makes you susceptible to bone fractures, in particular the spine and hips, and can cause you to look much older because of the hunch which may develop in your upper back and spine from the loss of calcium from your bones.

Walk with your shoulders and back straight, and put energy into each step. Concentrate on standing straight, even when not walking, which will keep your back muscles tense and consequently keep your bones healthy. Both you and your bones will look great as you walk away bone loss, and you will keep your figure looking beautiful.

Osteoporosis is a serious debilitating disease affecting over 20 million Americans, mostly women over the age of 50. This condition is actually a degeneration of bone throughout the body resulting in a loss of bone density. The bones actually become thinned-out as a result of a loss of the mineral calcium from the bone structure. Osteoporosis is especially marked after menopause because of a reduction in the secretion of estrogen by the aging ovaries.

Osteoporosis leads to approximately 1.5 million fractures each year. Fractures of the hips are particularly common in older women.

Approximately one out of every five older women who sustains a hip fracture dies of secondary complications. This results in almost 3,500 deaths every year, making osteoporosis a leading cause of death among senior citizens. Another 25% of these women who break their hips become permanently crippled. Other serious complications of osteoporosis are fractures of the spinal column. These fractures can cause a collapse of the spinal vertebrae resulting in a shortening of actual height, a severe curvature of the spine ("dowager's hump"), or a paralysis of the spinal cord.

There are many therapies that are currently undergoing investigation for the treatment of osteoporosis. Some of the treatments for osteoporosis include calcium supplements with vitamin D and medications designed to prevent bone loss. These and other recommended treatments have to be tailored to each woman, by her own physician. What do you think are the most important ways to prevent osteoporosis? *Walking and weight-bearing exercises lead to stronger bones and less chance of fractures.*

In a recent study reported in the *Journal of Orthopedic Research*, women who remained physically active after menopause or after age 50 had stronger, denser bones. Compared with inactive women ages 50-75, the active women had considerably greater arm and spine bone density measurements, almost in the same range as women 10-15 years younger. This study supports earlier research that shows that *osteoporosi*s (thinning of the bones) can be slowed or halted by a regular walking program combined with weight-resistance exercises, and that the incidence of bone fractures is ten times less frequent in these women. The **Power Diet-Step Walking Workout Exercises** and the **Diet-Step® Walking Plan** not only makes your muscles stronger, but they also stimulate the growth of the bones under the muscles.

Walking outdoors when the sun is shining also helps to strengthen bones, because sunshine helps the body produce vitamin D, a nutrient needed for calcium absorption. And, if these walking women ever do have the misfortune to break a bone – *their bones unite (heal) faster!*

The National Osteoporosis Foundation suggests four steps to prevent osteoporosis in both men and women:

1. A diet rich in calcium and vitamin D.
2. Weight-bearing exercises and walking.
3. No smoking and limiting alcohol intake.
4. Bone density testing supervised by your physician.

10 REASONS TO TRY WATER AEROBICS

1. Water aerobics burns approximately 400-500 calories an hour (based on a 140 pound person) and it's great for your bones and body.
2. Water aerobics won't make you sweaty.
3. This type of exercise is easy on your joints.
4. It improves balance and coordination.
5. Water aerobics tones every part of your body at once.
6. This activity allows you to control the level of difficulty at your own pace.
7. Water aerobics maintains a heart rate at a safe level.
8. This exercise provides a cardiovascular workout equal to land aerobics.
9. Water aerobics are less intimidating than land aerobics because no one knows if you miss step and you don't have to keep up with the instructor.
10. And most importantly, it's fun.

TIP #100
LOSE WEIGHT! LIVE LONGER!

Inactivity is associated with obesity, diabetes, hypertension, heart disease, pulmonary diseases, gastrointestinal disorders, arthritis, back problems, muscular and mental tension, and premature death. Walking, on the other hand, increases the delivery of oxygen to the brain and the body's tissues, which improves the circulation. This oxygen delivery results in increased energy and mental alertness. Walking also decreases stress and tension, thus producing muscular and mental relaxation. Walking lowers your blood pressure and helps to prevent cardiovascular disease by lowering the LDL (bad cholesterol) and the triglycerides (sugar fats) and by raising the HDL (good cholesterol) in your blood stream.

Walking burns calories, which helps to prevent and control obesity and diabetes. Walking builds muscle and bone tissue and helps to prevent osteoporosis, arthritis, and degenerative muscular and neurologic disorders. Walking prevents the development of chronic lung disorders by keeping the lungs and respiratory muscles in good working order, and by preventing the lung capacity from shrinking.

Walking boosts the immune system by producing chemicals known as *interferons* that do everything from warding off colds to preventing cancer. In fact, when you come right down to it, walking helps to prevent almost every known disease and disability known to modern science. And above all, walking helps to prevent premature death and even mature death. Walking will allow you to live many years beyond your predetermined genetic-coded death. Population studies show that *walkers live at least 10 to 15 years longer* than their sedentary counterparts.

Walkers in every country in the world have been proven to be the longest-living segment of any population of any civilization. From the Masai natives in Africa to the Russian tribes in Siberia; from the mountain climbers of Peru to the Bushmen of New Guinea; from the train-workers in London, England, to the mailmen and women of the United States, they all have one thing in common – *they're all walkers!* And for all intents and purposes, they live longer than any other similar-age group of people in their respective cities or countries.

Dr. Alexander Leaf, Professor Emeritus, Clinical Medicine, Harvard Medical School, studied varied populations throughout the world and concluded that the active segment of each population had a longer lifespan than the inactive segment. He stated – *"It is apparent that an exercise like walking throughout life is an important factor promoting well-being and longevity. One is never too old to commence a regular program of exercise and, once started, will never grow too old to continue it."* Walkers live longer and are illness-free longer than their sedentary counterparts anywhere in the world. This was the conclusion reached at the last national convention on Clinical Research on Aging.

In the majority of cases, obesity results from too little exercise and too much food. Life insurance studies have shown that excess weight causes cardiovascular disease with a significant increase in mortality. These same studies also reveal that life expectancy improves following weight reduction. Obese people have a significantly higher incidence of hypertension than non-obese persons. The excess body weight demands a higher cardiac output (pumping out blood) to meet the increased metabolism of an overweight body. This, in turn, causes the left ventricle chamber of the heart to gradually enlarge because of this extra workload. The combined effect of obesity, hypertension, and heart enlargement may eventually lead to heart failure and death. Weight reduction can lower both the systolic and diastolic blood pressures, if it is accomplished before the complications of heart enlargement and heart failure occur. These medical conditions must always be treated and monitored by your own physician.

Obesity also causes an alteration of the body chemistry and metabolism. The **blood-sugar** goes up dramatically with obesity, often leading to the development of diabetes. The **uric acid** in the blood becomes elevated, often leading to kidney stones and attacks of gout. Obese people have higher levels of **triglycerides** (sugar fats) and the **"bad" LDL cholesterol**. They also have lower blood levels of the "good" HDL cholesterol. These altered blood fats can eventually lead to severe coronary artery disease. These abnormal blood chemistries can be reversed to normal levels, if weight reduction occurs before permanent complications result. And if all these risks of being overweight weren't bad enough, here's more evidence that being overweight is dangerous to your health. *Obesity, just by itself, has been listed as an independent risk factor for coronary heart disease.* Newer data from the 26-year follow-up statistics in the *Framingham Heart Study* demonstrated that obesity, just by itself, was enough to cause a significant increase in the risk of coronary heart disease and premature death in both women and men.

ENJOY LIFE AND LIVE LONGER

In two studies reported in the September, 2004 issue of the Journal of the American Medical Association, it was reported that walking prevented older people from losing mental function as they aged and reduced their risk of developing Alzheimer's disease. These two studies showed that a moderate physical activity such as walking was all that was needed to prevent this mental decline.

One study involving over 2,200 men ages 71-93, found that those men who walked less than ¼ mile per day were twice as likely to develop Alzheimer's disease as men who walked more than two miles per day. In a related study involving over 15,000 women ages 70-81, it was found that those women who walked approximately 1 ½ -2 hours per week did much better on tests of mental function and thinking ability than inactive women. These two studies show that moderate exercise may reduce the brain levels of a sticky protein called amyloid, which can clog the brain's cells, causing mental decline and Alzheimer's disease. Walking can also increase levels of naturally produced chemicals that protect the brain's cells from aging and can help to increase the blood flow to the brain.

LOSE WEIGHT AND LIVE LONGER

To live a healthier, longer life and to win the war against obesity, you need only to heed these two simple and effective precepts. One is to regularly follow a **low-fat, high-fiber, lean protein diet.** The other is to follow a **regular aerobic walking exercise program** every day. These two easy methods of diet and exercise will effectively reduce your weight permanently, lower your blood fats and help to reduce your risk of hypertension, heart disease, strokes and certain forms of cancer. These two important steps will *add years to your life and life to your years.*

MEDICAL MANOR BOOKS® QUICK ORDER FORM

Postal orders:
  Medical Manor Books, 3501 Newberry Rd. Philadelphia PA 19154
Toll Free telephone orders:
  1-800-DIETING (343-8464)
Fax orders: 215-440-9255
E-mail orders: sales@medicalmanorbooks.com
Web site orders:
  www.medicalmanorbooks.com
  www.100bestweight-losstips.com
  www.diet-step.com
On-line booksellers:
  Amazon.com
  BarnesandNoble.com
  BooksAMillion.com
              <All major credit cards accepted>

The following books by Dr. Stutman are available from Medical Manor Books®

Title of Book		Price
100 Best Weight-Loss Tips (Cloth)	ISBN: 0-934232-20-2	$29.95
100 Best Weight-Loss Tips (Paper)	ISBN: 0-934232-19-9	$19.95
Diet-Step: 20/20 –For Women Only (Cloth)	ISBN: 0-934232-10-5	$25.95
Diet-Step: 20/20 –For Women Only (Paper)	ISBN: 0-934232-09-1	$15.95
Walk to Win (Cloth)	ISBN: 0-934232-08-3	$19.95
Walk to Win (Paper)	ISBN: 0-934232-07-5	$10.95
Walk Don't Die (Cloth)	ISBN: 0-934232-06-7	$18.95
Walk Don't Die (Paper)	ISBN: 0-934232-05-9	$ 9.95

COMING SOON:
•Power Diet-Step: 21-Day Power Weight-Loss & Fitness Plan
•Diet-Step: 30/30-For Seniors Only
•100 Best Fitness Tips